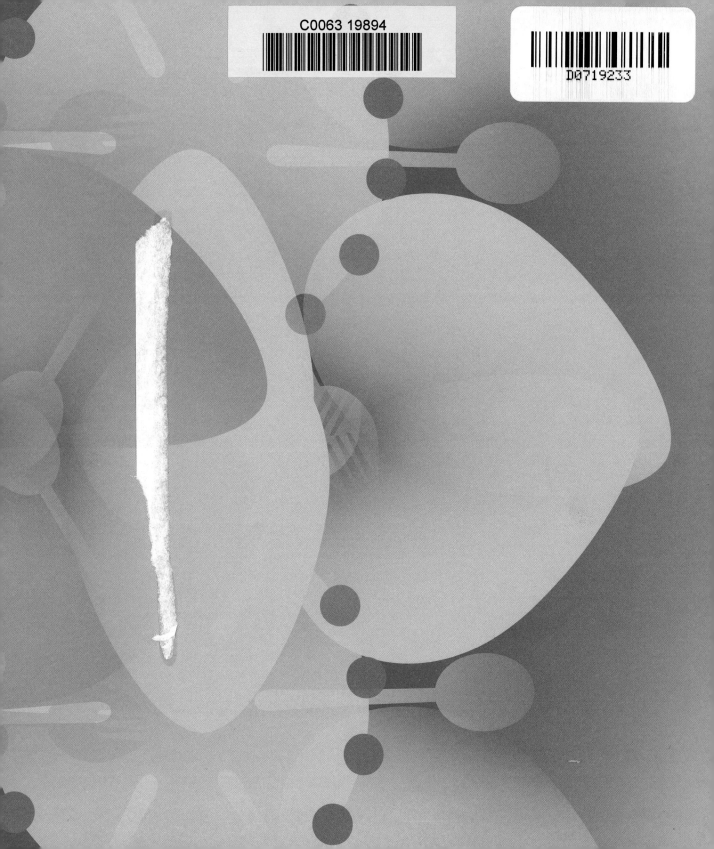

C0063 19894

D0719233

Everyday Strength

RECIPES AND WELLBEING TIPS
FOR CANCER PATIENTS

Sam Mannering
and Karen McMillan

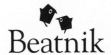

Beatnik

First published in 2017 by Beatnik Publishing

Text: © Karen McMillan 2017
Recipes: © Sam Mannering 2017
Photographs: © Sam Mannering 2017, with exception of page 214 & 215 © Sally Greer 2017

Design, Typesetting and Cover: © Beatnik 2017
Art Direction and Design: Sally Greer

This book is copyright. Apart from any fair dealing for the purposes of private study, research or review, as permitted under the Copyright Act, no part may be reproduced by any process without the permission of the publishers.

Printed and bound in China.

ISBN978-0-9941383-6-1

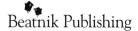

Beatnik Publishing

PO Box 8276, Symonds Street,
Auckland 1150, New Zealand

www.beatnikpublishing.com

Everyday Strength

RECIPES AND WELLBEING TIPS FOR CANCER PATIENTS

Sam Mannering
and Karen McMillan

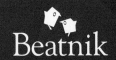

Beatnik

Contents

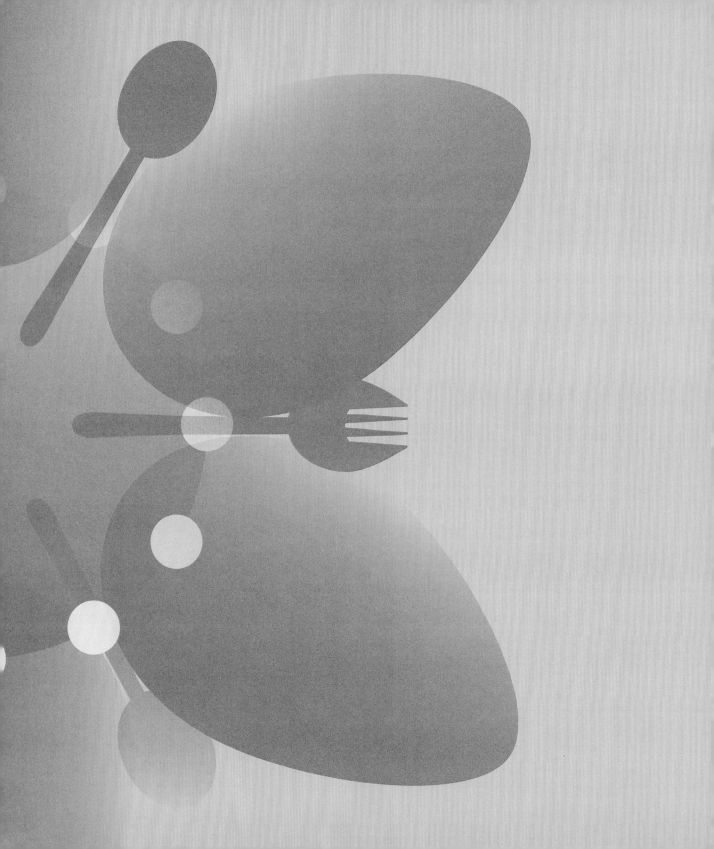

Preface

Together with acclaimed food writer Sam Mannering, Karen McMillan, the author of *Unbreakable Spirit*, has curated this innovative book that fills a void in the cancer and diet literature. It contains a quiver of sensible and practical tips for patients undergoing treatment for cancer. There are vignettes from patients for people to relate to. Within this book, you will find many recipes that will give patients and their support people ideas of what to prepare during this challenging phase in their lives.

Cancer and the various treatments required to maximise outcomes can often impact dramatically on dietary requirements and preferences – often in a deleterious way. I often get asked what foods patients should or should not be eating while undergoing treatment. This is difficult to answer as the best solution for an individual patient can be highly varied, depending on what the issues are and often an iterative strategy is required to establish what works best for each person. Patients will often be bombarded with advice including recommendations for radical diets, which may be based on opinion and which lack good evidence to support them. Furthermore such diets will commonly be less enjoyable in the context of someone's established dietary preferences.

Going through cancer treatment is a tough time in one's life and for most people, food still provides welcome enjoyment. For this reason it's important to eat foods they enjoy. Maintaining a steady healthy weight is also important and adjusting an individual's diet to enable this may be required (both weight loss and weight gain can be issues for patients with cancer). A healthy diet can ensure an adequate intake of vitamins and minerals, therefore preventing the need for yet more pills for supplementation. As detailed in this book, certain foods can be useful for ameliorating side effects of cancer treatment as well as reducing the need to take extra medicines for such problems (although these are readily available if needed – one just needs to ask). It is important to note however that dietary modulation should be seen as an adjunct to proven therapies to treat the cancer. It does not in any way replace evidence-based effective treatment.

Thank you, Karen and Sam, for giving those affected with cancer this comprehensive guide that will show how they might best negotiate their way through important cancer treatment. Not only will it fulfil nutritional needs but most importantly it will offset so much that is unpleasant with enjoyment through food!

Dr Reuben Broom
Medical Oncologist

How to use this book

The period of life when people are going through treatments for cancer has many challenges. This book is designed to help make each day a little better when someone is facing 'The Big C'. It is not a medical book, and it certainly doesn't promise to cure cancer, but it's been approved by medical people, and it has many helpful strategies, tips, and delicious recipes to make each day more bearable for those going through the different treatments for cancer.

Both Sam Mannering, the talented chef whose recipes are in this book, and myself are cancer survivors, and you can read about our personal stories further on. We have endeavoured to use our own experiences, but have also taken on board feedback from countless individuals and medical professionals to create a book that is full of the best and most practical tips to help you get through this most challenging of life experiences. This is not a book for the medical discussions you will be having at this time – you will need to talk to your key medical team about the questions you might have about surgery, radiotherapy or drug therapy (chemotherapy, hormone therapy, targeted therapy, immunotherapy).

*Rather, in **Everyday Strength**, you will find the lower-level, everyday things you can do to become more nourished from the food you eat so that you feel better and more optimistic. In short, we offer many small things that can make a difference and make each day a little brighter.*

There is no 'ABC' experience of cancer, of course, and inevitably, because we are all individuals, there will be a wide variety of concerns. Both Sam and I found that our concerns changed as we went through the forced march of our treatments. And because we realise this is a time when you can feel overloaded with information, this book is broken into common areas of concern that many people facing cancer may experience at some point or another. In this book you'll find sections on exhaustion, lack of appetite, or sudden weight gain. Matters such as nausea, reflux, diarrhoea and constipation, pain and discomfort are discussed. We tackle some of the typical symptoms of hormone therapy and we look at hair and skin care, as well as emotional wellbeing. And let's not forget the special section of recipes designed to tempt young children, along with practical tips for parents.

As well as evidence-based information, we have included opinions from a number of people on various subjects. These should not replace or negate the need for proven medical therapy. Details of some websites are also included for the individuals who have been interviewed here, so that you can learn more about the person/organisation if you are interested. Their inclusion is not intended to be an endorsement of their commercial activities.

As well as what we believe to be the best and most practical suggestions, this book contains many recipes, specially designed by Sam for all those dealing with cancer. **They all have an emphasis on being easy-to-prepare, nutritious and delicious – ideally suited for people who aren't well.** *In creating these recipes, Sam has taken into account the changes in individual palates – flavours that are warm and comforting, rather than the strong and spicy end of the food spectrum – typically experienced by people undergoing treatments.*

It's our hope that people will share this book, not least because many of the recipes can be made by friends and then frozen until required – a godsend for families at this time.

NUTRITION

Once you've been diagnosed as having cancer, you are likely to receive a lot of conflicting advice about your diet.

You may even look back at all the different foods you have eaten over a lifetime and start worrying that perhaps you ate too much charred meat and not enough spinach. But do be reassured on this score as there is no one food that causes cancer. In fact, the reasons why some people develop cancer are so complex, it's just not possible to single out one particular food as the culprit.

While dealing with cancer, try not to stress about the foods you are currently eating or think maybe you should be eating. Instead, try to eat a variety of foods that you enjoy, with an emphasis on whole food – ie, food that is as close to nature as possible, whether it be vegetables, fruit, meat, or seafood. We also recommend avoiding processed food – which you probably won't feel like, anyway.

The recipes in this book are a good starting point, as they are nutritious and feature fresh ingredients designed to be enjoyed by the whole family. Be moderate in your approach, and enjoy the nutrition that comes from each meal and snack.

IF IT'S YOU FACING CANCER

Being diagnosed with cancer is undoubtedly a difficult time and people will want to offer you help and advice. Stop, pause and consider what is best for you. We know that for some people the prospect of accepting assistance might be difficult, but you are going to need help to get through this time. Think about the kind of help you feel comfortable with, and allow people the privilege of assisting you. They really will want to help, so let them – but on your terms.

Listen to your medical team and, if in doubt, by all means get a second opinion. However, we suggest you trust their years of training and evidence-based studies a whole lot more than a quick information fix via the Internet. We also want you to be aware of all the support agencies that exist to help you at this time. You may be pleasantly surprised at what is available in your community.

Remember that it's up to you how private or public you want to be about your cancer journey – there is no right or wrong way, as it should be purely a personal choice. But whatever you decide, make sure you have the support you need. Now is the time to include your close friends and family and enlist their help if that is your choice, but do think about what assistance you actually want before you share with people. Here are some things to consider:

Nutritious meals

If you want meals cooked for you, share this book with friends and family and make them aware that many of the recipes here can be popped in the freezer. Tell people about the kinds of food you currently feel like eating. They aren't mind-readers and will be grateful to have some direction.

Practical help

Make a list of things that friends and family can do, eg housework, gardening, childcare, being driven to appointments, etc.

Pampering and nurturing

It's really important to treat yourself at this time so try to arrange visits from friends (when you are up to it), make time for reading, listening to music and going to the movies. A massage and similar special treatments are also really good for raising your spirits.

Contact person

Arrange for someone to be the contact point for updates; either via email, social media, text or phone calls. It's perfectly OK to use group emails, texts or posts in this situation.

People will tell you it is good to be positive, but it's also OK to have a good cry when you need it. You don't have to be brave every day. Feel what you feel and go with it. It is much healthier to accept whatever it is you feel than to fake it.

During your treatments, give yourself permission to be Number One for a while; you have to put yourself first to get through this. And if you feel you need to pay back your friends and family, you can do this when you are well again. It's not selfish; it is just making sure you don't run yourself more ragged than necessary.

IF IT'S SOMEONE YOU CARE ABOUT FACING CANCER

Understandably, people can feel unsure about what they can do in this situation. They don't want to intrude and they don't know what is appropriate. But remember your friend or family member is still the same person you know and love, so don't be frightened to make contact – you are only showing you care. Here are some tips:

Make contact

Drop them a note, email, text, post, tweet or phone message as soon as you can by whatever means is best for you both. Offer to help, but don't be pushy about rushing around to see them. Keep in touch on their terms.

When you visit

Let them talk about their concerns and be prepared to listen. Your role is not to be a fixer, so resist giving advice. By simply listening, you can help with their concerns. It may be that they will prefer to talk about everyday things, so try to sense their mood and be guided by it. Keep things real – it's OK to show your emotions, it's OK to admit that you're not sure what to say and it's even OK to have a laugh. Keep your medical opinions to yourself, however, unless you are a trained professional.

Respect their wishes

Never doubt that it is all about them. Whatever they want, try to go along with it – even if you don't fully agree with it. Keep reminding yourself that it is all about them. And as mentioned on page 10, practical help can be a godsend. Making meals, driving, babysitting, housework and gardening will mostly be really appreciated by a sick person. Do be aware that some people find it hard to ask for help, so don't be shy about offering to do something practical for them.

Gifts

Receiving a small gift or perhaps a bunch of flowers can lift someone's spirits when they are undergoing treatment for cancer. It really is the thought that counts, so there is no need to buy lavish gifts. Books, magazines, DVDs, CDs, hand cream and pot plants are good examples of thoughtful gifts. A copy of this book would also be appropriate.

Financial help

Personal costs often increase at these times. If someone's budget is already tight, things like hospital parking, transport costs, away-from-home accommodation and childcare can add to a family's stress. If it is appropriate, you may be able to pay for some of these costs. However, this will need to be handled sensitively, in order not to offend. Much will depend on how close you are to the person who needs help. And if it's not appropriate to offer financial assistance for whatever reason, then consider a gift card for petrol or groceries, either of which will be more helpful to them than a bunch of flowers.

Don't forget their partner

While most of the focus will be on the person with cancer, the person caring for them shouldn't be overlooked. They may also be going through a difficult time, and the caring suggestions listed here can equally apply to them.

Also, keep in mind that cancer treatment can be a lengthy process so it's important to keep in touch as time passes.

EVERYDAY STRENGTH

We hope people facing cancer, along with their friends and family, will find this book an invaluable resource at this difficult time, and that every day will be a little bit better by using the suggestions and recipes in these pages.

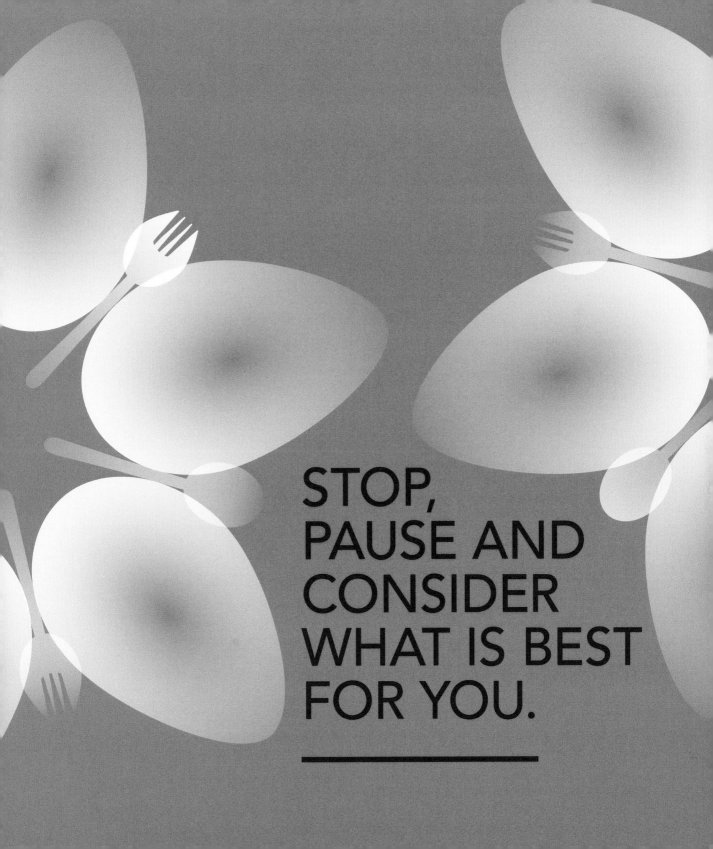

STOP,
PAUSE AND
CONSIDER
WHAT IS BEST
FOR YOU.

I WON'T DENY
HOW DIFFICULT
THIS WAS; TO LOSE
BOTH MY PARENTS
TO CANCER
STILL SEEMS
INCOMPREHENSIBLE.

_____

Karen's Story

Cancer has had a huge impact on my family. At the age of fifteen, and then for the next nearly fifteen years I experienced first my father and then my mother living with and ultimately dying of cancer in the prime of their lives. I won't deny how difficult this was; to lose both my parents to cancer still seems incomprehensible. I feel much sadness, but I also remember the times of love and laughter, and I'm grateful for the many lessons I learned from them. My paternal grandfather passed away after suffering throat cancer, and one of my mother's younger sisters had breast cancer, but is, thankfully, a survivor.

I became a volunteer for my local hospice after my parents died with the intention of wanting to give back after all the help that particular organisation had given me when caring for my parents. I've written many stories to promote the life-affirming work they do as well as interviewing those who were terminally ill, their families and caregivers and hospice staff. Interviewing Mitch Albom, author of *Tuesdays with Morrie*, was the catalyst for writing *Unbreakable Spirit: Facing the Challenge of Cancer* – a book of inspirational real life stories about people facing cancer, including the stories of both my mum and dad. I've since received so many beautiful

letters from families telling me how my book has helped them. As I had hoped, different chapters resonated with different families, but they all found useful aid and comfort from the various stories.

Since *Unbreakable Spirit* was first published cancer has struck my family again. One aunt with bowel cancer, an uncle with melanoma and a cousin with ovarian cancer. They have all survived. Sadly, though, my father's youngest sister's short battle with pancreatic cancer ended with her death at age 64. But cancer hasn't affected everyone in my family. My maternal grandmother died a couple of years ago, after a long and healthy life, at the age of 95.

In 2011 I faced my own battle with breast cancer, but mine is largely a positive story. It's a story of being informed and catching a potential killer early. It's a story of battling cancer with lots of support from my medical team, family and friends.

It's a story of faith and positivity. It's a story of a good prognosis, of being healthy and happy, and fully engaged with life again. But the forced march of cancer was undoubtedly hard – possibly the most difficult thing I have ever been through in my life – and certainly the most physically gruelling.

Despite my family's experiences of cancer, and interviewing scores of people with cancer, I've learned that nothing can prepare you for receiving the diagnosis yourself. I'd been in the habit of having annual mammograms and ultrasounds in my thirties, well before the recommended age. As I'd become a little blasé about these appointments, it was a huge shock in 2011 when I went for my regular appointment during which my breast physician discovered a lump while doing the ultrasound. It took a while for my brain to process the news, and after I'd had a biopsy a short time later I remember very clearly that I started to physically shake.

I received the biopsy result on a Friday, and on the following Monday my husband and I went to see the surgeon, who provided us with a number of well-considered options. This made it easy to decide on a mastectomy, especially as I was fortunate enough to be in the position where they could do a reconstruction at the same time. I remember feeling very calm about this decision, and soon afterwards we began to tell the people who needed to know.

In hindsight I think I had made a decision a long time before actually finding out that I had cancer that I would choose to be open about things if I ever found myself facing this particular life challenge. I have always thought that my father's model of telling everyone ended up being the better option than my mother's choice, which was to try to keep things extremely private. My father had his share of insensitive people, but overall the support and love he received far outweighed any ill-thought comment. As for myself, I felt being open would be easier in terms of getting the support I needed – and I thought it would probably be easier for the people who cared about me, too. People were obviously shocked but very supportive when they heard the news so that we were able to discuss that, yes, I had a frightening disease, and I was going to lose a breast, but I wasn't having a personality transplant.

We phoned my sister, who, understandably, was upset – she had already lost both her parents to cancer and now her only sibling had the disease? It was terrible news to share with her, but we were able also to tell her the positives: it looked like it had been caught early and it would be fixable. After that she made plans for when she would come to stay with us.

What I remember from this time, and indeed, the entire duration of my cancer battle, is how kind people were.

I am blessed to have such caring people in my life. So many flowers arrived at home it looked like a florist's shop. People also sent cards and small gifts and letters of support. Seemingly endless comforting messages were left on both our phones. I had dear friends all around the world praying for my health, as well as people from my church. I was truly overwhelmed by the genuine love and care from my friends and family – even from people I didn't know that well before I was diagnosed.

When the time came for surgery it went well, but the bad news was that the tumour was much bigger than we had expected: 5.3cm instead of 2cm. But the good news was that my lymph nodes were clear; one of the most important issues with breast cancer. And thanks to being able to have a reconstruction at the same time, there was something under the bandages; the beginning of my new breast.

My recovery after surgery also went well in that I was out of the hospital within three days and back to work in a few weeks. If having surgery was an important day, the next D-Day was getting the results a few weeks later. More good news in that the surgery had removed all the cancer, with close but clear margins. The results showed that it was an oestrogen-positive ductal breast cancer, too, also good news as there are drugs available to shut down one's oestrogen. But instead of the Grade One cancer we were expecting it was in the grey area of a Grade Two. This, coupled with my relatively young age, led to the

specialists meeting to discuss my case so they could recommend treatment options. It looked like I would have to do more than just undergo surgery, but it wasn't exactly clear at first what I would need to do next.

My husband and I attended a number of appointments to get the information we needed; I was adamant that after losing both of my parents to cancer I wanted to do everything possible to prevent a recurrence. I didn't want to be facing secondary cancer in five years' time – now was the time to undergo any preventative treatments.

Long story short, it was decided I would go through a three-month treatment of chemotherapy, five weeks of radiotherapy on my new breast and then I would go onto a drug called Tamoxifen. This was the same drug my mother had taken all those years ago – it would block the action of oestrogen (which was fuelling the breast cancer cells). Statistically, there was a good reason for putting myself through all of this. Post-surgery I had a 70 per cent chance of being cancer-free in ten years' time, but by undertaking all these treatments I could bump my survival statistics up to 86 per cent. I knew they would be tough, but I considered myself extremely fortunate to have these options. Far worse would be if I were told I had cancer, but that they couldn't do anything about it.

Chemotherapy was admittedly very daunting. My father had had a terrible time with it, but I was reassured by my wonderful oncologist that they had much better supportive care medicine now, so they would be able to mitigate some of the troubling side effects. I was scheduled for four treatments every three weeks. I did as much as I could to prepare for chemotherapy – I spoke to the people at my workplace and we established, in conjunction with my oncologist, what we thought would be a realistic work plan over that time. Then I had my hairdresser cut my hair into a short bob, plus I bought a wig. I was nervous, but ready to take on the challenge.

I opted to have my chemotherapy in the hospital ward with several other women, rather than going through the treatment on my own. It was a good decision as it turned out to be a surprisingly upbeat experience. The other women were very welcoming and happy to share their experiences, and we were soon sitting around and swapping stories like we had known each other for years. The nurses were wonderful, very professional and caring.

Each treatment cycle ended up being much the same – the feeling of being poisoned for the first week, which slowly got better by week two and three of the cycle, before heading into hospital for another round. I still have the drug information sheet with three pages of possible side effects for each, including nausea, vomiting, mouth ulcers, hair loss, diarrhoea, tiredness and feeling weak as just some of the common side effects. I've only recently gone through and marked off the symptoms I personally experienced. For the first drug, I had six of the possible side effects. For drug two I had seven of the possible sixteen side effects. So it was not too bad really. I found the extreme tiredness and my lack of appetite the hardest to deal with. Some women complained about putting on weight, but I struggled to eat during my treatment. Everything tasted of tin! My husband, who is a fabulous cook, just didn't know what to feed me. I even went off eating chocolate, a luxury I normally love. The only taste that I enjoyed during those months was balsamic vinegar.

During my second round of chemotherapy my hair fell out – in the space of 24 hours. It was very dramatic, but rather than being upset I found it fascinating. I got my hairdresser to shave off the remaining wispy bits and was then thankful to have my cute wig on standby.

It gave me the confidence to continue working (I didn't like the way my bald head identified me as a cancer patient). Then I decided to try to inject some humour into the situation when I felt well enough by wearing a cheap fun wig on our dress-down Fridays. A bright pink wig was one of my favourites. At home, though, I usually wore a beanie or left my bald head uncovered. My husband was very sweet and often told me that I had a lovely head and that I looked like a store mannequin.

My decision to work through my treatment was certainly a challenge. As hard as I tried, I just couldn't manage a full day; although most days I started work around 9am and worked through to about 4pm. Halfway through the treatment, I had to admit that I felt completely knackered, bald and beaten up. It didn't seem to matter how much I rested or slept; I just felt exhausted! I noticed one night that the skin on my face was flaking off as if I'd had a mild sunburn. At that point, I began to mark off the days on the

calendar like it was a prison sentence, with my last treatment date of 29 November highlighted. In the photos taken during my last chemotherapy session, I look tired but triumphant. I had made it through! But weeks later, when we broke up from work just before Christmas, I distinctly remember my feeling of total exhaustion; I felt like I was about 90 years old.

Radiotherapy was the next treatment on the list, and thankfully I tolerated it quite well – although I know some people find it tough. It was halfway through the treatment before my skin began to look a little burnt. By the end the affected skin looked horrific – the area was bright purple. But my skin stayed intact, and it wasn't actually as painful as it looked. Around this time my hair was growing back, and my husband said I looked like a little soldier with a short buzz cut.

On 1 January, 2012, I started taking Tamoxifen – fully expecting to have menopausal symptoms – but I was delighted to experience no real side effects, apart from drier skin and hair. At around this time I also got approved for a gene test to investigate the family history of breast cancer. After extensive research, it was decided that I didn't have a mutated BRCA gene 1 or 2 (like Angelina Jolie), but I put a

DNA sample on their files in case it would be useful to my nieces in the future.

It was time to start looking ahead, and my husband and I had already decided to book a five-week trip to Europe in mid-2012, with a plan to visit some of the best beauty spots. It was an incredible adventure for us as a couple, given everything we had been through during the cancer treatment; a time that was arguably just as hard on my husband as myself.

But I did listen to my GP's advice, despite the excitement of a dream trip. She warned me about not overdoing things for the next year. She knew I was keen to get back to the many things that I'd had to drop when going through my treatments. It was excellent advice. When we got back from holiday I caught every illness going around and in retrospect I found this to be the most difficult period, in terms of my emotions. I felt fragile, and not quite ready for everyday life. I lost confidence in myself – my body, my mind, my abilities. I'd been warned that feeling like this was very common, but it was hard to go through, and it took time for me to come out the other side.

I've had days when I've embraced the fear. Instead of my 86 per cent chance of survival, it was the 14 per cent statistic of not surviving that haunted me. My body had done it once, so why wouldn't my body do it again?

Some of the people I met during my treatment didn't do so well. Then there was the interview I did with a woman at my local hospice, younger than me, who was terminally ill with breast cancer. It was my first assignment after my recovery. She died two days after I interviewed her. A dear friend who was a huge help to me during my cancer battle moved to the UK – and later died. Given these connections it would be impossible not to have thoughts about my own mortality. The only way to combat the fear is faith. Faith in my medical team and that all the information they have told me is correct – but more importantly that all of it is in God's hands.

One of my aunties said I would be 'dangerous' when I had fully recovered – and six years on while I am well and healthy again I don't consider myself dangerous, although I have got my mojo back. I now have my own successful business, I'm still working in book publishing, and after a break of a couple of years I am back writing. Life is undoubtedly good, and I feel very blessed.

People ask me if having had cancer has changed me. I don't think you can go through having cancer without it changing your life in some way. My husband and I have always had a very close relationship, but we are now even closer. My faith in God is stronger. I feel older than I used to, in ways beyond that of my actual age. I am well, but I need more sleep than before and I don't want to physically push myself like I used to. I certainly feel more fear about matters such as illness and death in that should I get cancer again, it might not be so fixable next time. Interestingly, though, I find myself taking more risks in life, and I don't care as much what other people think. But by the same token, I want to give back more to the people and causes that are important to me.

*I hope that sharing my story will help other people facing their own cancer battles. I got through to the other side, and I trust that other people can also get through this challenging life experience with their spirit intact, ready to face the next stage of their life. And I also hope that **Everyday Strength** will be a valuable resource for people in the midst of their cancer treatments. It has so much information that I wish I'd known when I was in the middle of my own battle, so I hope that some of the tips and recipes included in these pages will help make each day for you a little bit easier.*

I THINK IN LIFE YOU HAVE TWO CHOICES. YOU EITHER DEAL WITH SOMETHING, OR YOU DON'T.

Sam's Story

Personable, young and talented, Sam Mannering is the author of several bestselling cookbooks, and he is also a regular food columnist and contributor to a variety of publications. When I started to think about finding a talented cook to create recipes for this book, he was my number one choice. The reason? Sam's recipes are among the most used in our kitchen because they are so delicious. He focuses on beautiful, fresh ingredients, and despite the restaurant-quality aspect of his meals, he creates dishes that are easy to prepare and which don't have a daunting list of ingredients. When I asked him to become involved in this project, he was immediately on board with the idea, and it was only after he had committed to the concept that I discovered that he is a cancer survivor like myself.

I caught up with Sam on a bright winter's day at Auckland's historic Pah Homestead, which houses not just a magnificent art gallery but also Sam's own well-regarded restaurant. After ordering tea we sat out on the large deck where we could enjoy the spectacular view and we talked about Sam's battle with melanoma, not once but twice. The most recent time involved removing cancer from the right side of his face, near the cheekbone and just under his eye. It was, potentially, a devastating thing to happen to a high-profile cook, who also treads the boards as an actor when he isn't creating in the kitchen.

'There's a small scar,' he says, pointing to his cheek. I look carefully but can't see anything. *'It's ironic. I have fair skin, so the scar only shows up if I get too much sun. The scar goes white, while the rest of my face goes beetroot.'*

We both agree it's a good reminder to stay out of the sun and then I settle back to hear Sam's story.

'My family has always been vigilant about doing mole checks. My grandfather, on my mother's side, died in his early sixties. My father's side of the family has fair skin, so they have needed to be careful, too. So getting mole checks has always been part of my consciousness.

'In my late teens I noticed a freckle on my thigh looked particularly dark, so I had it looked at. Within a week it was cut out, and I was gobsmacked just how far down they had to go to cut it out. I was only under a local anaesthetic, so I was sitting there, watching this take place. I don't get queasy or anything like that, but it was quite shocking to see how much they took out. So that was my first experience of melanoma.'

After this experience, Sam was even more vigilant, and it was part of his new routine to have regular checks, in some cases having suspicious-looking moles removed, all of which were, thankfully, benign. But in the winter of 2014, he noticed a freckle on his face had suddenly blown up.

'When this freckle flared up on my face, I went to my doctor and had her look at it immediately. She was concerned and took a scraping.'

Sam was prepared for bad news when he went back to the doctor. It was soon apparent that he had another melanoma to deal with – this time on an extremely visible part of his face. But he chose to take this news in his stride. And although his parents were overseas when it happened, he drew on lessons he'd learned from them.

'I think in life you have two choices. You either deal with something, or you don't. It's a lesson I've learned from my family. I know it's easier said than done, but I consciously decided to deal with this. Of course, we are all human, and it's okay to feel emotion at this terrible news, but I was determined to carry on living my life like before.

'I didn't deny the cancer or the reality of having to do treatment, but I accepted this was my new reality and that it was something that I had to deal with. I also didn't want to give the cancer any more power than what it already had, and I consciously chose to live my life, as much as possible, as though I didn't have this new knowledge.'

Sam had intensive radiotherapy for most of the winter of 2014, while juggling the demands of producing his second cookbook, *Food Worth Making.*

'I'm a firm believer in keeping busy, and I've usually got many projects on the go. It makes life exciting, so I didn't want to give up creating the new cookbook. But I was lucky as this was my own project which I could do in my own time. It probably would have been different if I had been working for someone else during this period, which is the reality for a lot of people. So I had flexibility that others might not have.'

Sam admits that the radiation was not only painful, but a claustrophobic experience. He also had terrible bruising during the treatments, but he was able to find the humour in the situation, despite presenting a different face to the world.

'I didn't go out much during this time, but when I did, I used to put on a hat and dark specs to try and hide the effects of radiotherapy. My flatmate and I used to joke about my new look. I sometimes get dark bags under my eyes, but during the treatment, I looked like a panda!'

Like me, Sam was amazed at how much sleep he needed while he was going through the treatments.

'I'm a farmer's son and before this, I thought anything past 6am was a sleep-in, but my body just demanded sleep. I know it seems ridiculous, but I'd go to bed at 3pm and wake up at something like 11 the next morning. I would watch a movie, or do a little bit of work on the new book, and that was it.'

As the melanoma was so close to the cheekbone, there was some concern it might metastasise, but Sam has been given the all clear. I ask him if he worries about the cancer returning.

'I get a little bit nervous sometimes when I see a freckle come up, but I keep a vigilant eye open. I go for regular checks. I've got one on my chest at the moment that I need to check. But getting checks is just part of my life now. And it affects my family, too. Dad has had a couple taken off already. And my sister and my aunt have had a few removed. It's a family thing, and we just need to deal with it.'

I ask Sam if his experience of cancer has changed his attitude to food, as it is so clearly an important part of his life as a professional cook. While he admits that he went off a few things like red meat, tomatoes and chillies while he was going through treatment, he says his overall view of food hasn't changed.

'Given our farming background, we were all very straightforward about food. I always ate what was on my plate, that is just what you did. When I went to boarding school, it was the same thing. For me, food is about being rational and intelligent, and it helps to have an understanding where food comes from and what has been done to it. For me, food is not just a way of satisfying hunger. Food is much more. It nourishes, it keeps you happy, and it uplifts you.'

And does he feel differently about the areas from which he has had the melanomas removed? It turns out not so much about his leg, but his face is a different story.

'It's had an effect on how I feel about my face. It is hardly noticeable, but there is still a weird awareness of it. It feels different. Even touching it now, this side feels different. There is a numb sensation. I suppose it's just scar tissue; it's just one of those things.'

While Sam fought hard to keep life going as normally as possible, he says it was a time of self-discovery.

'By going through this, you work out what your strengths and weaknesses

are. It's like starting a business or being in a relationship with someone; going through something as life-changing as cancer, you start to see a lot about yourself that you have never really thought about before, things that you haven't necessarily been confronted with. It's a make or break thing, and you have to react to it. I've learned a lot about myself.'

At the time I first wrote about Sam's experiences both of us thought this chapter was done and dusted. But then I met with him many months later into this project – for one of our regular meetings – and Sam delivered a bombshell. He had just been diagnosed with his third melanoma – this time on his left hand.

'I'm very lucky that it was in a place where I could see it. I immediately saw my GP who is a skin expert. Samples were taken, and within a couple of days, I had the news that this was a melanoma. I've since had it cut out, and I've had two radiotherapy sessions on it.'

Sam admits that he was initially stunned by the news as it had been a very busy year for him. Overwhelming, in fact. He had been looking forward to the Christmas holidays and heading to the beach and relaxing.

'I was stunned this was happening for the third time, and I would have to have treatment again. I had a boys' night out soon after my diagnosis with some of my very good friends, and I think that is when it hit me. We'd had a few quiet drinks after dinner, and one of my friends was opening up about his brother who had died of MS. I think that's when my situation caught up with me. But I am lucky, my specialists had never said it was serious, and we caught it before it had a chance to spread. Of course, it's natural to worry, but it's a bit like getting into a car and thinking it will lead to a car crash. I just viewed the whole thing as a process. I'm thankful it has healed quickly.'

I was so impressed by Sam's positive approach. Although I could tell he was a little shocked by another diagnosis of melanoma, he immediately saw it as a positive for writing this book. Once again he was back facing the hard reality of the Big C, and this helped him to create the many wonderful recipes in this book – recipes created with care and insight of what it is like to be at the coalface, going through treatments, and not quite feeling your usual self.

Finally, I ask him if he has any advice for others facing cancer.

'Cancer is a hideous thing, but I think it helps if you have an attitude of trying to make it as pedestrian and ordinary as possible. I believe that you shouldn't give it more power than

it deserves regarding who you are and your life. Cancer could happen to anyone, so I wouldn't spend time being bitter or vilifying it. But you do need to confront it and do what you think is right when you are facing it. For me, it helped to live my life as normally as possibly while going through treatment.

'Telling my story now is about context and a platform for positivity. I hope this book will enable others to live their lives in a positive way when facing cancer.'

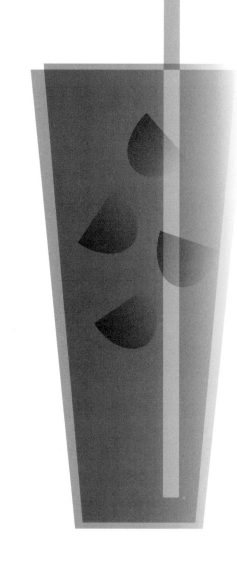

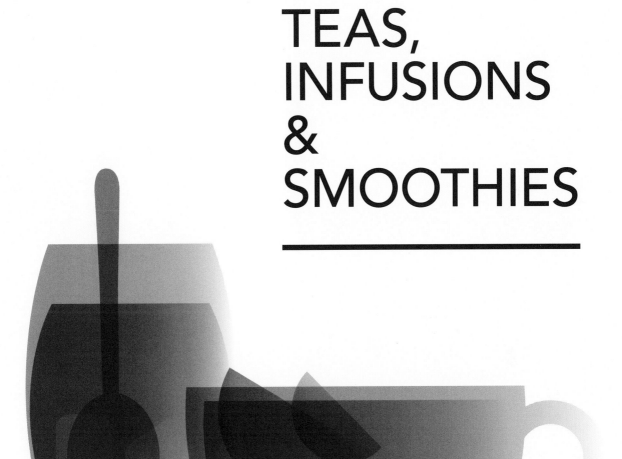

TEAS, INFUSIONS & SMOOTHIES

Infusion for a Cold

1–2 PREP: 5 min COOKING TIME: 15 min GF DF

INGREDIENTS:

4 slices fresh root **ginger**

1 **cinnamon stick**, broken in half

2 **whole cloves**

1 tsp **coriander seeds**

½ **lemon**, sliced

500ml **water**

manuka honey

In a saucepan bring the first 6 ingredients to the boil and simmer gently for 15 minutes. Strain and sweeten with manuka honey to taste. Add a good slug of whisky for a grown-up infusion. Note: this is also very soothing to drink if you have a sore throat.

Gargle for Sore Throat

1 PREP: 2 min COOLING TIME: 10 min GF DF

INGREDIENTS:

2 tsp dried **sage**

1 tbsp **cider vinegar**

1 tbsp **manuka honey**

1 cup (250 ml) **boiling water**

Combine all the ingredients, set aside to cool right down, and then strain. Use to gargle with several times a day.

Moroccan Mint Tea

◯ 1   PREP: 2 min   INFUSION TIME: 4 min   ✿ GF   ◉ DF

INGREDIENTS:

fresh mint

brown sugar

1 cup (250 ml) boiling water

Per person, take a generous handful of fresh mint, on the stem and combine with boiling water in a tall glass or mug, and leave to infuse for 3–4 minutes. Add enough brown sugar to taste.

Lemongrass and Ginger Tea

◯ 2+   PREP: 5 min   INFUSION TIME: 4 min   ✿ GF   ◉ DF

INGREDIENTS:

1 large thumb fresh unpeeled ginger

2–3 stalks lemongrass, fresh or frozen

juice of ½ lemon

1 tbsp honey

Cut the ginger into 3–4 slices, each about 0.5cm thick and crush them with the flat of a heavy knife. Cut the lemongrass in half lengthways. Combine all the ingredients in a teapot and top up with hot water. Leave to infuse for 3–4 minutes.

Blueberry, Coconut and Lemon Smoothie

 1   PREP: 5 min   COOKING TIME: 2 min   GF   DF

INGREDIENTS:

½ banana

squeeze of lemon juice

1 cup (100g/3.5oz) blueberries

2 tbsp coconut cream

200ml almond or regular milk

Blend until smooth.

Kiwifruit, Mint and Honey Smoothie

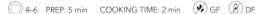 4–6   PREP: 5 min   COOKING TIME: 2 min   GF   DF

INGREDIENTS:

1 kiwifruit, peeled

½ banana

2–3 mint leaves

1 tbsp honey

200ml almond or regular milk

Blend until smooth.

Banana, Cocoa and Cinnamon Smoothie

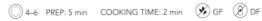 4–6   PREP: 5 min   COOKING TIME: 2 min   GF   DF

INGREDIENTS:

1 banana

1 tbsp **cocoa powder**

1 tbsp **honey**

½ tsp **ground cinnamon**

200ml **almond milk**

Blend until smooth.

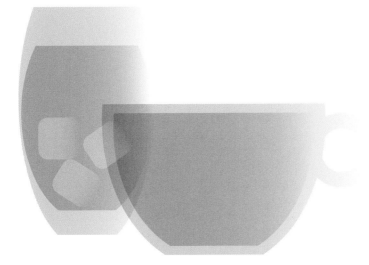

Exhaustion

PRACTICAL SOLUTIONS FOR THIS COMMON PROBLEM

'In general, chemo makes you feel like you have a constant combo of jet lag and a hangover. You get very sick and tired of feeling sick and tired.' – Lindsey

'I was told I would get a bit tired having radiotherapy. Tired? It's like suddenly switching off a light bulb; you are absolutely exhausted' – Sinda

Exhaustion is probably the most common symptom experienced by those facing cancer. Prevalent and distressing, fatigue can occur during treatments and for some people, fatigue can persist for anything from five to ten years after diagnosis. For anyone facing cancer, this is certainly a symptom you will, if at all possible, want to minimise.

NUTRITION

Good nutrition is a key factor in combatting the fatigue associated with cancer, and the recipes in this book will go a long way towards improving energy levels. I spoke with Wendy Hamilton from Optimum Health & Nutrition and we discussed the importance of proper nutrition at this time. A registered nurse and a respected natural health practitioner, Wendy has excellent advice about your diet while facing cancer.

'A big thing to consider is keeping your blood sugar levels balanced because that has an enormous contribution to energy in the body. So for anyone facing cancer, or even just wanting to look after their health, my message to them would be to eat real whole food.

'By that I mean, natural foods, primarily plant-based food, accompanied by protein sources of food such as nuts, seeds, legumes, eggs and good quality meat. These foods release their nutrients gradually and will help your energy levels.'

Wendy advises people to avoid as much as possible foods that have been processed or which contain chemicals and sprays. She also recommends staying away from food with high levels of sugar, which can lead to feeling even more exhausted. Looking after your adrenal health is another important factor.

'Stress and poor food choices tire the adrenal glands. The way to eat to support the adrenal glands is to balance blood-sugar levels. When the blood sugar is going up and down like a roller coaster, every time the

blood sugar comes down into the low sugar range, the adrenals get called and can go into "flight or fight" mode. So the benefits come from eating steady meals. Try eating a snack or a meal every two and a half to three hours, which will stop your energy from dipping. Keep up the energy level by fuelling the tank steadily through the day. While you may not want to eat big meals when going through cancer treatment, it's good to keep the nutrients coming in, so you just don't dip and get exhausted. That's why having snacks is a good idea if you can't face a big meal.

'At every meal and every snack you should eat good quality carbohydrates such as vegetables and fruit, with some protein of some kind. That could be either animal protein or vegetable protein such as nuts and seeds. Every meal or snack combo should have both these elements, which are valuable for energy.

'You could also consider removing foods from your diet, to which you might have a sensitivity. The most common ones are gluten and conventional dairy. I often hear that people's energy just soars when they come off these things.

'Smoothies are an excellent option at this time. Make them using predominantly vegetables, with just one serving of fruit to make it pleasurable. You might even want to add some seeds and nuts, as they will add fibre, minerals and good oils.

'If you have three meals a day along with some snacks, why waste those opportunities to fuel your body? Put an emphasis on making everything count, which means eating nutritious and healing food. Because, as Hippocrates said, that is what food can do: "Let food be thy medicine, let medicine be thy food."'

All the recipes in this book will help minimise exhaustion, so enjoy the good nutrition that will come from every well-balanced meal and snack.

DIGESTION

Healthy digestion plays a significant role in your energy levels. And the easiest way to help your body digest food? Make sure you chew it properly. Give your digestive system a helping hand by chewing your food slowly. As a general rule, think 20 chews per bite.

HYDRATION

Are you drinking enough water? Dehydration fuels tiredness so it's even more important to keep your fluids up when you're going through cancer treatment. As roughly 70 per cent of your body is water, feeling dehydrated will impact on nearly every part of your body: your blood, your lungs, your brain, your muscles, even your bones. Ensuring a regular intake of water is crucial for energy.

Herbal teas and soups will also contribute to your overall daily water consumption. And as many fruit and vegetables comprise over 70 per cent water, the more you can eat of these the higher your water consumption will be.

Wendy Hamilton has this to say about the importance of water in our diet, along with enough good salt.

'Drinking steadily through the day is important; 30ml per kilogram of body weight is a good water calculation. Eight glasses daily is an average for most people, but it's best to avoid alcohol and coffee if you are unwell. Herbal teas, though, are a great idea as consumption of them will increase your overall water consumption. Green tea is high in anti-oxidants, ginger tea is fantastic because it's anti-inflammatory and good for nausea, peppermint tea helps digestion and lemon juice in hot water is good, too. Try to find a nice herbal tea that you like, one that will comfort, boost your immunity and help your condition.

'Good salt is also essential as salt in the body helps water move to the right tissues. I recommend an unbleached Celtic sea salt, or a Himalayan mineral salt – half a teaspoon a day with eight glasses of water is very good.

'On the subject of drinking water, make sure it is purified, filtered water if possible. There are relatively inexpensive filter systems that will be cheaper than buying bottled water all the time.'

WISCONSIN GINSENG

In a trial led by the Mayo Clinic in 2013 Wisconsin Ginseng (Panax quinquefolius) a common type of American Ginseng, showed good results in helping cancer patients with fatigue, when compared with a placebo. The conclusions of the study supported a daily dose of 2000mg of American ginseng to improve cancer-related fatigue, with no discernible toxicities associated with the treatment.

It should be noted that on this trial there wasn't a great improvement after four weeks, but at the eight-week mark there was a sudden jump in the general energy levels reported by the group taking the ginseng. It would seem the herb takes a while to work its magic, but those taking the ginseng supplement found their general exhaustion diminished rapidly at this point.

Ginseng is a slow-growing perennial plant with fleshy roots, and while there are eleven different varieties, the two major species are American and Asian. A smaller study reported positive effects of Asian ginseng in patients receiving chemotherapy. Ginseng has been touted for centuries as a trusted herbal remedy, useful in boosting energy, lowering blood sugar and cholesterol levels, reducing stress and promoting relaxation. Note that the quality of the ginseng is important. If you are interested in taking ginseng I recommend that you discuss it with your oncologist.

SLEEP

Sleep is your best friend when you are going through treatment for cancer as it gives your body a chance to repair and recover. Don't be alarmed if you find you need many more hours of sleep than the traditional eight hours. This is perfectly normal. Naps are also OK. But if you are struggling to sleep, here are some tips that may help.

Look carefully at your bedroom. Consider your bed in particular – is it old and uncomfortable? Now might be the time to consider purchasing a new bed. Look also at your pillows and duvet covers. Comfort is especially important now, so replace old bedding if possible.

Keep the room cool and dark and remove all unnecessary electronics. Is your alarm clock causing you stress? Do you find yourself glancing at your clock during the night, feeling increasingly anxious that you are still awake? Put your alarm clock in a drawer or turn it away from view.

Are you experiencing mild pain? Your lower back may not hurt enough to wake you up, but mild pain can disturb the deep, restful stages of sleep. Put a pillow between your legs to better align your hips and place less stress on your lower back. Do you sleep on your back? Tuck a pillow under your knees to ease any pain.

Are exterior noises keeping you awake? Try using ear plugs, or turn on a fan or air conditioner to create 'white noise' to mask traffic or other noise that might be keeping you awake.

Do you allow pets on your bed? Consider banning them while you're undergoing treatment if they are keeping you awake. But if your pet is a huge comfort at this time, as many are, you may prefer that they are on the bed with you. Clearly, it is over to you, but remember that you have to do what is best for you. Your pet's needs at this time are secondary.

Establish a soothing routine before bedtime. An hour or so before you intend going to bed choose a calming book to read, meditate, listen to quiet music, or take a warm bath.

Taking a melatonin supplement may also help. Melatonin is a man-made form of a hormone produced in the brain that helps regulate your sleep and wake cycle. Talk to your doctor about this option or perhaps sleeping pills if none of the other suggestions work for you.

EXERCISE

When you are undergoing treatment, it can be easy to think you are too tired to exercise, even when gentle, appropriate exercise is recommended. I highly recommend making an effort, though, as exercise boosts metabolism, increases oxygen in your blood and releases endorphins, all of which will give you a mental boost.

I met with Lou James, a physiotherapist who founded the PINC & STEEL Cancer Rehabilitation Trust (an Australasian cancer rehabilitation movement founded in 2005) to learn about the work they do with cancer patients. Their philosophy is to look at the whole person when recommending a rehabilitation plan and they believe exercise is important for minimising exhaustion.

'Any surgery and treatment will impact on your body, so it's important to see a physiotherapist to be assessed. When you know what you can do, not only does it improve your recovery and increase your energy levels, it is also empowering that you can help yourself.'

If you have surgery or other treatment scheduled, Lou recommends you see a cancer rehabilitation physiotherapist as early as possible.

'They will assess you and then they will put a plan into place for you, with all the tips and things that can help you stay as well as you can during this period. They will look at how your body is moving and functioning and will work with you to get your body functioning normally again. They will discuss with you what you want to get out of it.'

Research has shown that if you exercise during chemotherapy and related treatment, you are more likely to finish your treatments. But forget your old work-out routines; exercise needs to be gentle and appropriate to your circumstances.

'It's all about listening to a person's body, and that's where a good physiotherapist can advise someone who is dealing with cancer. Often you do need to rest and recover, but exercise will help to invigorate you and give you more energy. Like when you feel sick, and you go for a walk, and the sun is out, and you feel a lot better. It's the same thing with what we do; people leave the clinic feeling better. We are talking very gentle, controlled stuff that can make you feel better and help get you through a tough time.

'One of the biggest effects of cancer treatments is deconditioning fatigue and exhaustion, and lack of energy. And that is not a normal tiredness, it is all-over body exhaustion, which affects every aspect of your life. You can't do the things you like to do as you are feeling so terrible. So any bit of improvement you can get in your energy levels and being able to sleep and function better is a massive help.

'Consider it like this. If you were going to run a marathon, you would want a coach supporting and guiding you while you were training for this physical challenge. Cancer is one of the biggest challenges that people can face. You need someone to help guide you through those treatments as they are extremely tough.'

Lou tells me that it's not possible to give general guidelines on what type of exercise is appropriate for people going through treatment as they prefer to do it on an individual basis. But she did stress that any exercise needs to be gentle – especially for those who were active prior to being diagnosed; they can't just expect to do their usual work-out routine.

'It's impossible to give a general guide about what exercise to do as it is going to vary so much; it depends on your age, your fitness level before you had cancer, and the kind of treatment you're having. Some people can't cope with as much exercise as other people, but everyone can do something. Our organisation has physiotherapists working in palliative care and even in hospice people are exercising. So you can do things to feel better, but it just needs to be very individually driven. As a general rule, it is reduced exercise in intensity and frequency.

'But it becomes a problem when people get told they should exercise, so they try to do what they did before, which for example, might be an hour's walk around the hills. But it's too much at this time, and then, when they feel terrible, it just adds to their feeling of exhaustion. Using this example, a person might go for a ten-minute walk and come back feeling good. And maybe another short walk a couple of days later. But it would be sensible to avoid steep hills, and instead perhaps drive somewhere to meet with a friend and then walk along the beach. It's important to get the right advice about exercise, and to think about the intensity and the terrain and how you are doing things.

'It is empowering when people can exercise a little bit. It gives them some sense of control. Often when someone is going through cancer, their control is taken away from them. Gaining some control back is mentally and physically a good thing. I would say to families and friends of someone with cancer to try to help them with the rehab side of things. Go with them to their physiotherapist, find out what is suggested so you can support them. It's about finding out what they need, rather than saying, "Oh, I don't think you should do anything today." Understandably, people can get very protective, so

finding out what exercise is appropriate and encouraging them is helpful.'

I ask Lou if it's possible to say how often people might expect to see a physiotherapist, but she tells me that like exercise, it's very much an individual matter.

'There is no typical scenario. Some people sail through surgery, others have a lot of complications, and they need help with scar management and pain. So it might take four or five sessions, or it might be more. Exercise is like a prescription, and a physiotherapist will help you get the right amount at the different stages of the cancer battle.

'It's also about being active in a way you enjoy. If you have never gone to the gym, it doesn't mean you have to start now; there are lots of options. You aren't going to do it if you hate it. If you are more comfortable exercising in your home, a physiotherapist can give you some appropriate exercises. I was talking to a colleague the other day who told me that someone they were treating ended up doing ten minutes of dancing to their favourite music each night. It's about choosing things that are going to make you feel good.

'But you do need to be realistic about what you can do. One of my patients was training *for a half marathon when she found she had breast cancer. She had the idea that although she'd missed that event, she'd do the next one! I didn't want to crush her enthusiasm, but I wanted her to be realistic. For people who have been very active, it is difficult for them to pull back on their work-outs. But exercise does put stress on the body, as does chemotherapy along with other cancer treatments, so you have to use exercise to invigorate you, not to add more stress. It's about taking rests. One of my patients said to me that she allowed herself to have a "pyjama day" each week, a day when she didn't get out of her pyjamas. Full-time rest is not good for you, but you have to allow yourself to rest and recover.'*

A cancer rehab physiotherapist can help with fatigue management, which is especially important when people finish treatments and begin to go back to their regular lives.

'People tend to think that once their treatments are finished they will be able to go about their lives as before, and that may not necessarily be the case for a while. I think fatigue management is about managing people back to their lives. People forget that work is a stress, that having lots of visitors is tiring, exercise is tiring, so if you have all those things

on one day, then it is too much. So fatigue management is managing people's weeks, that is their activities and prioritising what is important, delegating what is not. For some people that is not easy to do, because they want to do it all. But this is a time they need to look after themselves. I think exercise is a priority, but don't then try to cook dinner for ten people that night. You have to learn to delegate things! Give your friends and family something practical to do that will help you as you ease back into your life.'

To access a cancer rehab physiotherapy service, ask your GP for a referral. You can find more about the PINC & STEEL programmes online.

EMOTIONAL STRESS

Worry can make you feel more exhausted – and having cancer can be an emotionally stressful time, with many uncertainties. Try to find an outlet for expressing your worries.

This might be through keeping a journal, sharing how you feel with someone close, art therapy, or losing yourself in music.

By sharing your anxieties with someone else, or by tackling how you feel in some creative way, it's possible to reduce the anxiety you feel. Let things out!

A never-ending to-do-list can be draining at the best of times, but even more so when you're facing the challenges of cancer – especially if you are juggling the demands of work and home life. Make a list of everything that needs to be done at work or home, then prioritise the tasks to see what is achievable. Delegate everything you can. If your workplace load is too much for you, do talk to your boss before things get worse. Most workplaces will be very accommodating in these circumstances.

In general, remember that it's OK for you to say 'no' when things get too much for you.

HOW TO GET HELP

When you are facing cancer, do get the help you need to get through this period of your life. Now is the time to call on friends and family – don't end up becoming even more exhausted trying to do all the things you used to do. Accept that it is just not possible and reach out for the help you need.

Sinda, who for many years worked for Sweet Louise, an organisation supporting people with secondary breast cancer, has had a cancer diagnosis also. She has many useful tips for getting the help you need based on her own experience.

'I'm an organised person, so even before surgery I had quite a few meals in the deep freeze, and I had this roster of people providing meals and soup. It was just fantastic. They organised meals that I liked over this period. People do like to help! For me, the meals were a big thing.

'I ate more vegetarian food during this time – that was just a personal choice. I started having cold pressed vegetable juices delivered. That way I didn't have to engage with anyone; I just put my cool box outside, and they put it in there and took away the empties. That was that!

'Be kind to yourself. The days you feel shocking, well you just feel awful, you can't make it better by going shopping. It won't make you feel better, in fact, it will probably make you feel worse. Think you'll go and sit in the café and admire the view? You probably won't even want coffee, so there is no point doing that. But you have to do things that bring you pleasure. I found browsing magazines was good because you can just pick them up and put them down again as you feel like it.

'If you can't do very much, get your support person to delegate jobs. People want to help, so by giving them something to do they are much happier. For example, ask someone to make a cottage pie for dinner. Even if they are

only asked once, it helps both you and them.

'I declined to have people drive me to appointments. But when I declined the offer I told the person that I'd get back to them if the situation changed. That's an important thing, people knowing you will come back to them if needed. It's OK to change your mind – your situation might change.'

So whether it is help with meals, housework, gardening, being driven to appointments or a babysitter for your children, don't be shy about asking for assistance. People want to be there for you, so let them help. That way you can concentrate your energies on your recovery and doing the things that will uplift you – not the routine stuff that may wear you down.

SOUPS

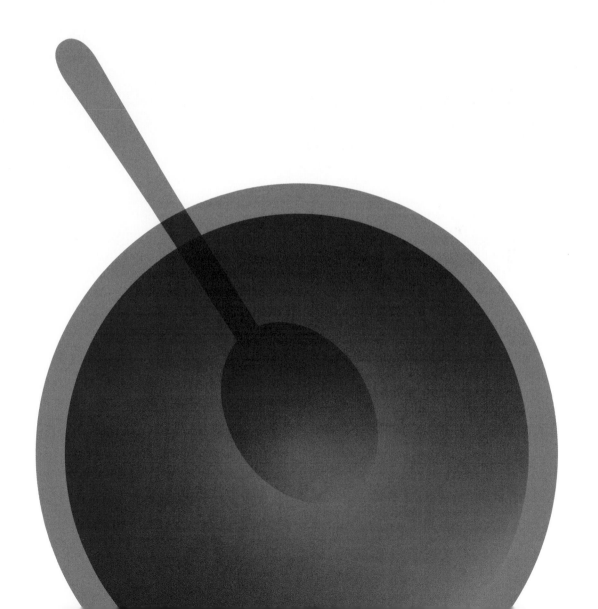

Pumpkin, Coconut & Lemongrass Soup with Vietnamese Mint

4–6   PREP: 10 min   COOKING TIME: 30 min   DF

INGREDIENTS:

1.5 kg (52.9oz) peeled and deseeded **pumpkin**, chopped into chunks

1 **red onion**, peeled and quartered

salt and **pepper**

vegetable oil

1 tsp **cumin seeds**

1 tsp **coriander seeds**

thumb-size piece **ginger**, peeled and finely chopped

3 tbsp grated **lemongrass**

1 **red chilli**, deseeded and finely chopped

handful of **coriander**, stalks included, finely chopped

handful of **Vietnamese mint**, chopped

2 tsp **fish sauce**

1 tsp **soy sauce**

400ml **coconut milk**

1 litre decent **vegetable stock**

½ cup (125ml) **coconut cream**

fried shallots, to serve

Preheat the oven to 180°C.

Spread the pumpkin and red onion out on a roasting tray, season well, drizzle generously with oil and give the tray a bit of a shake so that everything is coated. Roast for 20 minutes or so until the pumpkin is just tender and a little bit caramelised.

In the meantime, get a large saucepan going over a moderate heat. Add a little oil, let it heat up, and then add the cumin and coriander seeds and gently fry them for 30 seconds or so until fragrant. Add the ginger and lemongrass to the pan and fry for a minute or so to coax the flavours out, taking care not to let it burn. Mix in the chilli, most of the chopped coriander and half the Vietnamese mint, the roasted pumpkin and red onion, the fish sauce and soy sauce, coconut milk and stock. Bring everything to the boil and let it simmer for several minutes. Take off the heat and set aside to let it cool a little. Using a stick blender, carefully purée the mixture until it is nice and smooth. Alternatively, use a food processor or blender, but make sure it cools down somewhat beforehand so that it doesn't splatter everywhere. Taste and adjust seasonings accordingly. It may need a little more chilli, fish sauce or soy sauce, depending on your taste.

Serve with a little spoonful of coconut cream, some fried shallots and the remaining coriander and Vietnamese mint over the top.

Karen: Coconut milk is highly nutritious as it contains fibre, vitamins and minerals. And as it is lactose-free, it's suitable for anyone who's lactose intolerant.

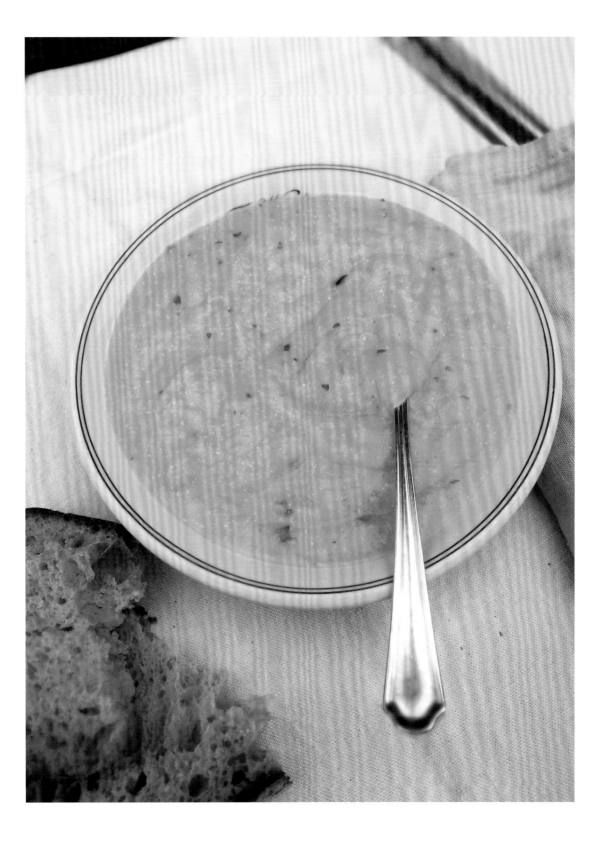

Spiced Chickpea Soup

4–6   PREP: 10 min   COOKING TIME: 30 min   GF

INGREDIENTS:

olive oil

1 **onion**, finely chopped

4 cloves **garlic**, finely chopped

2 tsp **ground cumin**

2 tsp **ground coriander**

1 tsp **turmeric**

½ tsp **ground cinnamon**

2 x 400g (14.1oz) cans **chickpeas**, drained and washed

1 litre **vegetable or chicken stock**

salt and **pepper**

natural yoghurt, to serve

handful of **coriander leaves**, to serve

In a large saucepan over a medium heat add about 1 tablespoon of olive oil and let it heat. Add the onion and garlic and cook gently for 8–10 minutes until soft, translucent and a little caramelised. Add the cumin, coriander, turmeric and cinnamon, and fry gently for another minute or so until the spices are nicely fragrant. Take care not to let it burn.

Add the drained and washed chickpeas, then follow with the stock, and bring everything up to a steady simmer. Let it bubble away for about 20 minutes or until the chickpeas have softened and absorbed the flavour of the spices.

Season well with salt and pepper, and serve with a little natural yoghurt and coriander served on top.

Karen: Little round balls of goodness, chickpeas are a wonderful vegetarian-friendly source of protein.

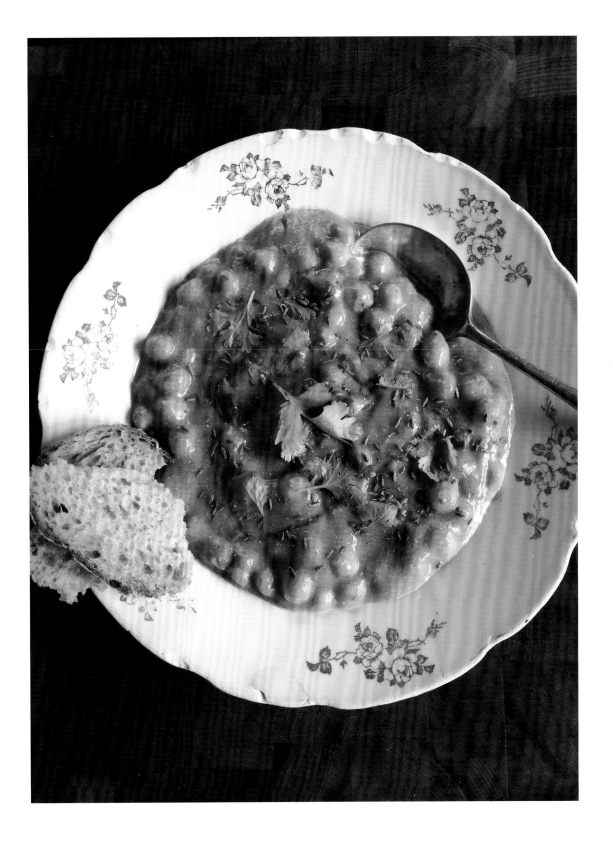

Rosemary & Cauliflower Soup

4–6   PREP: 5 min   COOKING TIME: 30 min   GF

INGREDIENTS:

2 tbsp **butter**

1 **onion**, finely chopped

sprig of **rosemary**

1 **cauliflower**, cut into florets

750ml **chicken** or **vegetable stock**

salt and **pepper**

½ cup (125ml) **cream**

Melt most of the butter in a large saucepan over a medium heat.

Add the onion and cook until soft and translucent. Add the rosemary and cauliflower and cook for several minutes, adding a little more butter if necessary. Stir in the stock, then cover and simmer for about 25 minutes or until the cauliflower is tender. Remove the rosemary and discard.

Transfer the mixture to a blender, in batches if need be, and purée until smooth. Return the soup to the saucepan and bring to a low simmer. Season to taste with salt and pepper, and add the cream to taste – about half a cup should do it.

Serve immediately.

Sam: This may seem a little basic, but as long as you season it well it is an absolute poster child for 'simplest is best'! Sometimes I like to add a little smoked fish to make it a bit more substantial.

Karen: Cauliflower is a particularly good source of Vitamin C. It has also got Vitamin B6, minerals and is a great source of fibre.

Ham Hock, Pea and Mint Soup

4–6   PREP: 5 min   COOKING TIME: 60 min   GF

INGREDIENTS:

1 tbsp **butter**

1 **onion**, finely chopped

3 cloves **garlic**, finely chopped

1 large **floury potato**, peeled and chopped into smallish pieces

1 whole **smoked ham hock**

1 litre **chicken** or **vegetable stock**

3 cups (450g/15.8oz) **frozen peas**

handful of **mint leaves**, finely chopped

salt and **pepper**

In a large saucepan over a moderate heat add the butter and let it melt and bubble up. Add the onion and garlic. Cook gently for 8–10 minutes until soft, translucent and slightly caramelised. Stir in the potato and continue to cook for 5 minutes. Add the ham hock, frying it gently on all sides, then add the stock. Bring everything up to a gentle simmer, then leave to cook for about 35–40 minutes or until the meat is falling off the bone and the potato is very soft. Add the peas and cook for another 10 minutes, then gently stir in the mint and allow to simmer for a final 5 minutes.

Remove the ham hock from the pan and when it is cool enough to handle, pull all the meat off the bone. Return the shredded meat and the bone, back to the pan.

Season to taste, and serve.

Karen: This a beautifully delicious and nutritious soup – perfect comfort food!

Lentil, Cumin and Silverbeet Soup

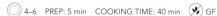 4–6   PREP: 5 min   COOKING TIME: 40 min   GF

INGREDIENTS:

200g (7oz) **red lentils**

olive oil

1 **onion**, finely sliced

2 cloves **garlic**, finely chopped

1 stick **celery**, finely chopped

2 tsp **cumin seeds**

1 tsp **sweet paprika**

½ tsp **cinnamon**

1.5 litres **chicken** or **vegetable stock**

salt and **pepper**

large handful of **silverbeet**, washed and sliced

plain yoghurt, to serve

Wash the lentils and drain well.

In a large saucepan over a moderate heat, add a generous glug of olive oil and let it heat up a little. Add the onion, garlic and celery and fry gently for about 6–10 minutes until it is soft and translucent. Stir in the cumin, paprika, cinnamon and drained lentils and continue to cook for another 2–3 minutes. Add the stock, then leave to simmer away quietly for about 20 minutes, stirring occasionally, until the lentils are soft.

Season well to taste. Stir in the silverbeet and cook for another 7–8 minutes.

Serve with a dollop of plain yoghurt on top.

Karen: Red lentils are packed with nutrition, making this a great recipe for taste and with health benefits.

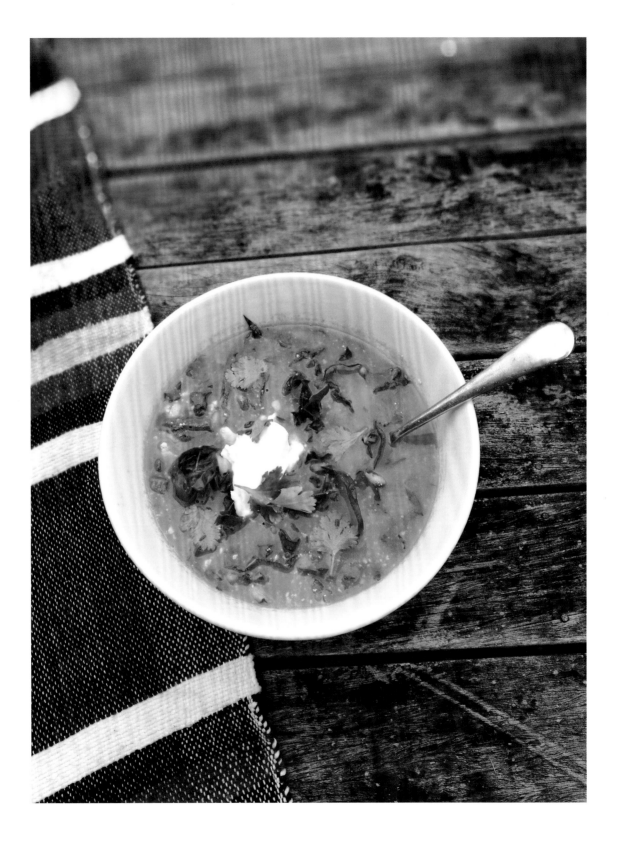

Onion and Thyme Soup

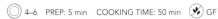 4–6   PREP: 5 min   COOKING TIME: 50 min   ✿ GF

INGREDIENTS:

1 tbsp **butter**

2 large **onions**, finely sliced

1 large **potato**, peeled and roughly chopped

several sprigs of **thyme**, plus a little extra

1 litre **chicken** or **vegetable stock**

salt and **black pepper**

½ cup (125ml) **cream**

Melt the butter in a large saucepan. Add the onion and cook very slowly for about 20 minutes until soft, golden brown and nicely caramelised, adding more butter if necessary. Add the chopped potato and continue to cook for several more minutes, then stir in the thyme and stock and a generous amount of seasoning to taste. Simmer gently for about 25–30 minutes or until the potato is soft and starting to break apart.

Fish out the thyme stalks and discard, then purée the mixture using a stick blender or food processor until smooth. Return the soup to the saucepan and add the cream and more salt and pepper to season. Serve with a few thyme leaves sprinkled over the top.

Karen: With among the highest antioxidant concentrations in any herb, thyme has been praised for thousands of years as an overall health booster. Sprinkle some true goodness over this superb soup.

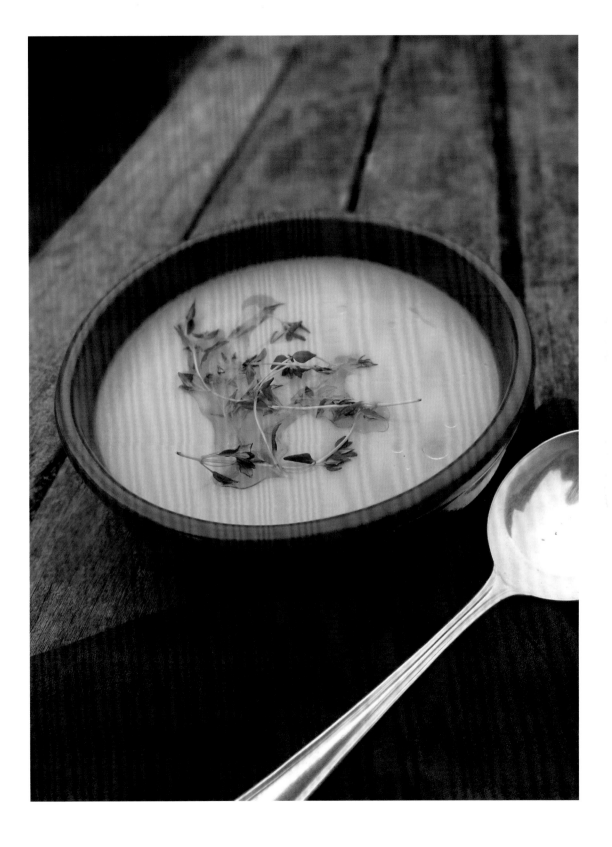

Lack of appetite and weight loss

'I struggled to eat during my cancer treatments. Food had no appeal, and everything tasted awful. But I persevered with different flavours, and eventually found some recipes that worked for me.' – Susan

'I discovered that eating small and often was the best solution to my lack of appetite when I was having chemotherapy.' – Tina

Lack of appetite can be a very real problem for many people facing cancer, especially those going through chemotherapy who tend to find that most foods, even their favourites, taste like tin. The most common aversions seem to apply to sweet foods, some fruits, particularly citrus, meat, spicy and strong-tasting foods, eg tomatoes and onions. It's also usual for people to go off alcohol and coffee. Note that these are short-lived food aversions and once chemotherapy is over you will go back to enjoying the foods you did before. Be aware also that changing your diet to accommodate the change in your taste buds while you're undergoing chemotherapy shouldn't have a major effect on your weight and nutritional intake.

A lack of appetite and subsequent weight loss is particularly problematic for people who are in palliative care, however. Michelle Kean, Household Manager at Hospice North Shore, was kind enough to meet with me and also to give permission to adapt some of their invaluable suggestions for this book. What follows is practical advice for anyone who is struggling with their appetite.

Eating and drinking are part of everyday life, so eating and drinking with family and friends can help you to feel better emotionally, which can improve your quality of life. And here's a lovely tip: try listening to music to relax you while you eat.

Eat small amounts, presented attractively.

In many ways, we eat with our eyes, so make your food appealing. Very small amounts of food on an attractive small plate can seem less daunting to try to eat than large amounts of food on a large plate. Arrange the food to look appealing on the plate. Add chopped parsley or snipped chives to create interest. Set the tray or table with some thought, add a flower or something beautiful to look at.

You may find using a teaspoon, rather than an ordinary spoon, is easier for you. And don't drink large amounts before or with a meal as it may make you feel too full too quickly. Take time to enjoy your meal and feel good about what you have eaten. Eat slowly in a relaxed environment, and chew your food well.

Eat frequently.

Forget about having three main meals a day, with your largest meal at night. Spread your food and eating times evenly throughout the day. Aim to eat breakfast, morning tea, lunch, afternoon tea, dinner and supper. Even if it's only a small amount of food each time, overall the amount you eat through the whole day will be greater. Eating like this is important as it stimulates the gut and can help it work better.

Aim to eat a variety of foods during the day. Try one new food at a time. If a particular food upsets you, perhaps try it again later.

Choose foods that are easy to eat. A sore or dry mouth can make some foods hard to chew or swallow, so try soft or 'melt in the mouth' foods that are easier to swallow. For main meals, cut meat, poultry, and vegetables into very small pieces and cook them with plenty of liquid until they are very tender, which will make eating and swallowing easier. Added gravies and sauces will also help. Soft milky puddings and ice cream can be good dessert choices, which you could even drink with a straw.

If you have trouble swallowing, it may help to use a thickener. Generally this is a starch-based powder that can be diluted in any liquid to give a suitable texture to make swallowing easier. Nutilis by Nutricia, or a similar product, is recommended as you can add it to drinks, puréed food, and nutritional supplements. It has optimal amylase-resistant features to ensure thickened food and fluid will maintain the prescribed consistency and not turn back to liquid in the mouth.

Eat the food you feel like when you feel like it.

Throw out the rule book! If you don't feel like eating a particular food, then don't eat it just because you think it might be good for you; try something you like better.

If your energy levels are low, don't wait until the end of the day to have dinner. Eat your main meal at lunchtime or when you feel least exhausted. Remember, too, that a light meal in the evening will be easier for your body to cope with during the night.

ALCOHOL

While the data on alcohol consumption is controversial, the general view from the medical professionals I spoke to is that a small amount of alcohol is OK. And if it is allowed with your drug and treatment programme, you shouldn't feel like you have to cut it out, especially if you would usually enjoy a drink. Alcohol stimulates the appetite and is a source of energy. It also makes you relax, which can help gut function, and a small amount may also help sleep. In fact, if you usually drink alcohol, it will probably help you to feel 'normal'.

FOODS TO AVOID

As a general rule, the foods you are probably best to avoid are:

- Spicy foods, curry, chilli

- Acidic food and drinks, raw tomatoes, citrus fruit, pickles

- Rough, tough foods (eg hard toast, dry cooked meat, raw fibrous vegetables such as uncooked cabbage and celery), and grapefruit and tamarillos

- Very hot or very cold foods.

Small frequent amounts of both food and drink are often better tolerated when you feel nauseated – try just a teaspoon or a sip at a time. Eat and drink slowly.

Cool foods are best at these times – jelly, cold desserts and ice-cream (although for some chemotherapy regimens you need to avoid cool foods – check with your oncologist). Cool drinks also tend to go down more easily – try diluted fruit juice and sports drinks. Also flat ginger beer or ginger ale. And don't overlook the benefits of sucking on an ice-block or some ice-chips.

Try rinsing your mouth or brushing your teeth with a soft brush before and after eating to make your mouth feel clean and fresh.

Another tip to make you feel better is to open a window or turn on a fan to keep the air smelling fresher.

ALTERED SENSES

It's very common for your sense of taste and smell to change when undergoing cancer treatment. You'll also find you could be nauseated by smells that would normally not bother you.

To make life as comfortable as possible:

- choose foods that do not have a strong smell, eg try cold ham, egg or chicken sandwiches or salads

- eat foods at a cooler temperature than usual (try lukewarm rather than hot) to reduce their aromas

- cool foods such as ice-cream, jelly, dairy food (all from the chilled section of the supermarket) have little smell

- keep away from the kitchen when food is being cooked if the smell puts you off eating.

Try different flavourings to help stimulate your appetite, eg lemon juice, fresh herbs, chutney, cheese, pepper, flavoured salt, soy sauce or balsamic vinegar. Many of Sam's recipes have been developed specifically to combat lack of appetite and weight loss. Our recommendations include:

- Pumpkin, Coconut & Lemongrass Soup with Vietnamese Mint, page 46

- Rosemary & Cauliflower Soup, page 50

- Moroccan Chicken with Preserved Lemon, Kumara and Spiced Yoghurt, page 104

- Roast Pork Leg Stuffed with Courgette and Garlic, page 110

- Curry of Pumpkin, Snake Beans, Cashews and Curry Leaves, page 112

- Tarragon Chicken, page 114

- Omelette Arnold Bennett, page 118

- Clafoutis, page 152

- Pear and Chocolate Crumble, page 162

- Chocolate and Almond Brownie, page 168

- Rice Pudding with Stone Fruit, page 178

Nausea

SIMPLE REMEDIES THAT MAY HELP

'Even though modern-day anti-nausea medication is very good, I still had days when I felt nauseous, much like morning sickness during pregnancy. The same strategies from back then – plain food to munch on – helped me through these periods.' – Amy

'I cleaned my teeth three or four times a day to achieve a cleaner sort of feeling. I sucked little mints, and a friend of mine who did chemo relied on boiled sweets. I tried crystallised ginger, too, in a bid to overcome the sour, metallic taste in my mouth.' – Lindsey

Smell is an important factor to consider if someone is experiencing nausea while undergoing treatment. If possible, keep cooking smells behind closed doors, away from the person suffering nausea. And avoid strong-smelling household cleaners. As a general rule avoid anything artificial smelling. Even scented candles may be a problem during this time, so replace them with those without an obvious scent. However, fresh light smells of lemon or mint may be tolerated.

Make sure you keep your fluids up to avoid getting dehydrated. Take frequent sips of water if you find drinking a whole glass at a time too much. A good idea is to make up a thermos of ginger root-infused or mint-infused water. Not only are ginger and mint both great for digestion and settling the stomach, they are also pleasant tonics to sip on.

You will probably want to modify your diet if you are battling nausea, and here are some tips that may help you:

Small meals and snacks. You might not feel like eating, but try five or six small meals instead of three larger meals. This will balance your blood sugar levels so are less likely to feel sick. Try to have some food before you go for any treatments – you are less likely to feel ill this way. Avoid fried, spicy, sweet or salty foods. Plain foods such as crackers or toast may help tame your tummy.

Think cool. Cool foods and drinks, such as jellies, yoghurts, desserts, flattened ginger ale or ginger beer can work well. Also eat foods at a cooler temperature than usual to reduce their aroma. Lukewarm is usually better than hot.

Here are some other tips:

- Ginger, whether in the form of ginger ale (the real stuff, not flavoured ginger), tea, or even raw, is proven to help control nausea. It promotes the secretion of various digestive juices/enzymes that help neutralise stomach acid, plus it contains phenols that relax stomach muscles and act as a sedative on irritated stomach tissue. Include ginger wherever possible in drinks, soups, smoothies and main meals.

- Peppermint is another aid to help combat nausea. Try sucking on a peppermint or chewing a stick of peppermint gum. Peppermint can relax tight muscles in your stomach and help decrease the stomach contractions that may be causing your nausea. Peppermint tea can soothe the stomach, while peppermint oil is excellent for digestion.

- Fresh mint added to salads and smoothies can make them more palatable.

- Place a few slices of lime or lemon in a plastic bag and freeze them. These slices are great to suck on if you are feeling nauseous and you don't have any fresh lemons available. As the smell of lemon can help you feel better, so too can the sharp, fresh flavour of lemon or lime in your mouth.

Then there are essential oils, which have many useful therapeutic properties, including reducing nausea. They should only be used externally, however, as they can be toxic if ingested. When applying essential oils to the skin, first dilute them with a carrier (olive oil, coconut oil, macadamia oil or rosehip oil all make great carriers). Try one or more of these three simple combinations:

> 2 drops ginger + 1 drop lemon in 5ml carrier oil. Inhale or gently massage over stomach.

> 2 drops peppermint + 2 drops lemon in 5ml carrier oil. Inhale.

> 2 drops peppermint + 1 drop ginger in 5ml carrier oil. Inhale or gently massage over stomach.

Acupressure wristbands may also help reduce nausea. How they work is that the wristband exerts pressure on the p6 acupuncture point on the wrist, which can relieve nausea and vomiting. They can be worn for as long as required.

Digestive enzymes, which can be purchased at a pharmacy, can also be helpful. They help the stomach to keep moving and not being 'locked up' by facilitating the chemical breakdown of food into smaller, absorbable components, which can help combat nausea.

Consider also how you manage any anxiety you may be feeling. Sometimes your fears about throwing up can be your own worst enemy. Simply acknowledge the thought and then let it go. And remember that getting out into the fresh air can help significantly. Gargling and cleaning your teeth are other simple things you can do to make you feel better.

If you do end up vomiting at any time, make sure you rest until you feel better. Then, after vomiting has stopped for an hour or so, sip some form of rehydration drink to restore lost fluids, eg weak tea or clear broth. Avoid orange juice, grapefruit juice, tomato juice, milk products, alcohol and carbonated drinks at this time.

Many of Sam's recipes have been developed specifically to combat nausea. Our recommendations include:

- Moroccan Mint Tea, page 31
- Lemongrass and Ginger Tea, page 31
- Kiwifruit, Mint and Honey Smoothie, page 32
- Ham Hock, Pea and Mint Soup, page 51
- Tarragon Chicken, page 114
- Pear and Walnut Gingerbread, page 156
- Bircher, page 180

SALADS

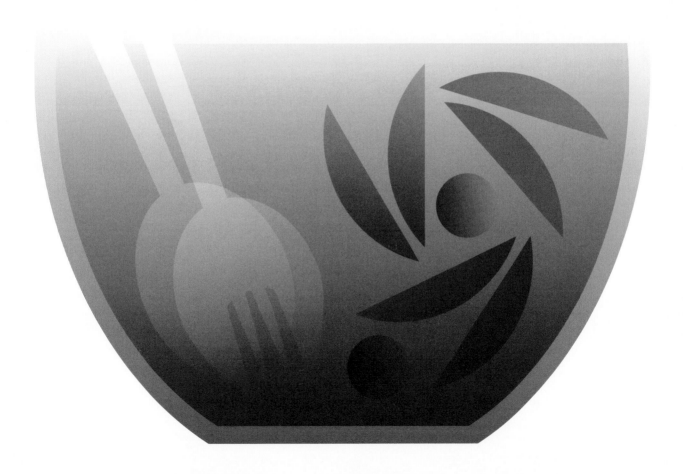

Salmon, Buckwheat, Fennel, Capers and Dill

4–6   PREP: 10 min   COOKING TIME: 15 min   GF   DF

INGREDIENTS:

200g (7oz) **whole buckwheat**

1 tsp **salt**

2 tbsp **olive oil**

zest and **juice** of 1 **lemon**

1 tbsp **Dijon mustard**

1 tbsp **capers**, roughly chopped

400g (14oz) **salmon fillet**, pin-boned

1 **fennel bulb**, cored and finely sliced

flaky sea salt and **black pepper**, to taste

small handful of **dill**, finely chopped

Place the buckwheat in a large saucepan along with the first measure of salt and add enough water to cover the buckwheat by at least 2cm. Bring to a slow boil and let it simmer away for about 10 minutes. In the meantime, slice the salmon as thinly as you can. In a wee bowl whisk together the olive oil, lemon juice and zest, mustard and capers with a grind of black pepper and toss together with the salmon and fennel. When the buckwheat is tender but not soft, take off the heat, rinse and drain well. Return it to the pan and let it heat up again in a little more olive oil, stirring so that it doesn't catch. When the buckwheat is nice and hot, remove from the heat and transfer to a serving plate. Fold the salmon and fennel mixture carefully through the hot buckwheat. Taste and season accordingly. Scatter the dill over the top and serve.

Sam: Buckwheat is a great vehicle for flavour. I don't like salmon to be cooked too much, which is why I like to thinly slice it in its uncooked state and then just fold it through the hot buckwheat (this gently takes the raw edge off). Alternatively, if you like it to be a little more cooked, just roast the whole fillet with a bit of olive oil, salt, pepper, lemon juice and zest on top. Gently flake the cooked salmon and then fold it through the buckwheat. If you don't want to use buckwheat, pearl barley is good, as is orzo, fregola (dot pasta), and Israeli couscous.

Karen: Packed with fibre and antioxidants, buckwheat has many health benefits, including being excellent for digestive health. Despite its name, it is completely gluten-free.

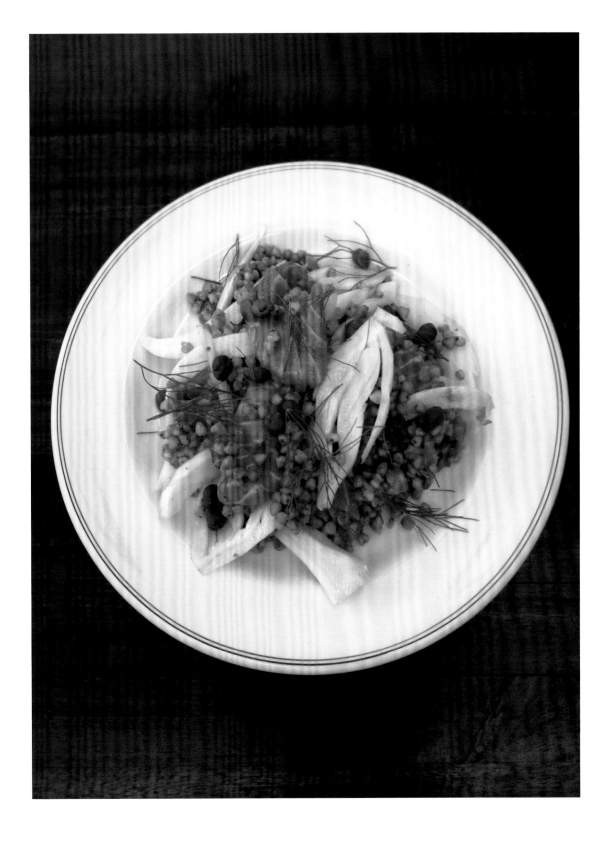

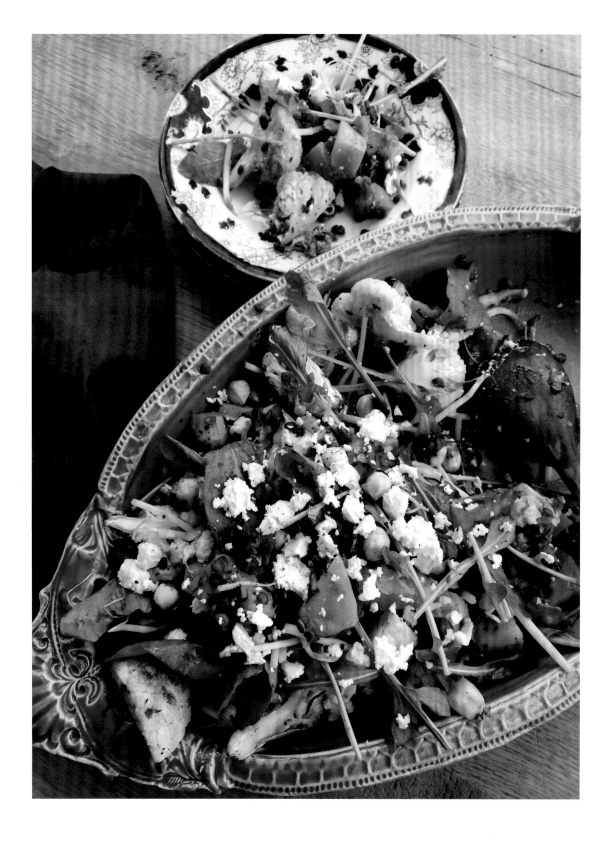

Salad of Pumpkin, Lentils, Cauliflower and Hazelnuts

4–6   PREP: 10 min   COOKING TIME: 40 min   GF   DF

INGREDIENTS:

½ crown **pumpkin**, peeled and deseeded

1 small **cauliflower**

sea salt and **black pepper**

olive oil

400g (14.1oz) **green** or **puy lentils**

handful of **bean sprouts**

½ cup (75g/2.6oz) **hazelnuts**, toasted and roughly chopped

large handful of **rocket**

Preheat the oven to 180°C.

Chop the pumpkin into smallish 3–4cm chunks. Remove the stem and leaves from the cauliflower and cut into florets. Combine both on a roasting tray with some salt and pepper and several tablespoons of olive oil. Shake the tray a little to coat the vegetables. Pop in the oven to roast for about 25–30 minutes until the vegetables are tender and nicely caramelised. Remove from the oven and allow to cool for several minutes.

In the meantime, wash and drain the lentils, then place in a saucepan with plenty of water. Bring to the boil, then leave to simmer gently for about 15 minutes until the lentils are tender. Drain off any remaining liquid, season well to taste with salt and pepper, and set aside to cool down.

On a large serving platter gently fold together the cooled pumpkin and cauliflower, the bean sprouts and hazelnuts with a little bit of olive oil and a generous seasoning of salt and pepper. Fold through the rocket and serve.

Karen: I'd say this is the perfect 'comfort' salad, if there is such an expression. Perfect for the whole family, but especially good for anyone undergoing cancer treatment as it's packed with nutrition and goodness.

Mushrooms, Roast Cauliflower, Pearl Barley, Walnuts and Feta

4–6   PREP: 10 min   COOKING TIME: 30 min   GF

INGREDIENTS:

1 **cauliflower**, cut into florets

a few sprigs of **rosemary**

olive oil

salt and **pepper**

400g (14oz) **pearl barley**, washed

500g (17.5oz) **mushrooms**

1–2 tbsp **butter**

juice of ½ **lemon**

handful of **rocket**

½ cup (62g/2.1oz) **walnuts**, toasted and roughly chopped

200g (7oz) **feta**, crumbled

Preheat the oven to 180°C.

Spread out the cauliflower pieces on a roasting tray and scatter the rosemary over the top. Drizzle with olive oil, season with salt and pepper and bake for about 30 minutes until the florets are tender, golden brown and slightly caramelised.

Place the barley in a saucepan with plenty of salted water and cook for about 25 minutes until tender, but not too soft. Drain and set aside.

In the meantime, slice the mushrooms. Get a saucepan going over a moderate heat and add a good tablespoon of butter. Gently cook the mushrooms in the butter until they are soft and fragrant, adding more butter if necessary as you cook them.

In a large bowl fold together the mushrooms, barley and cauliflower and drizzle in a little more olive oil and a squeeze of lemon juice. Taste and season accordingly. If you want to serve it as a warm salad, allow it to gently warm through in the oven before folding in the rocket, walnuts and crumbled feta.

Sam: This is a lovely way of using mushrooms – use a mixture of whatever varieties you like. Pearl barley is a joy to use – cooked until al dente, it helps to carry the other flavours and adds a good substantial element to the dish – as well as being incredibly good for you.

Karen: Mushrooms are magnificent for your health. They contain selenium, potassium, Vitamin C and iron, and are also a great source of protein.

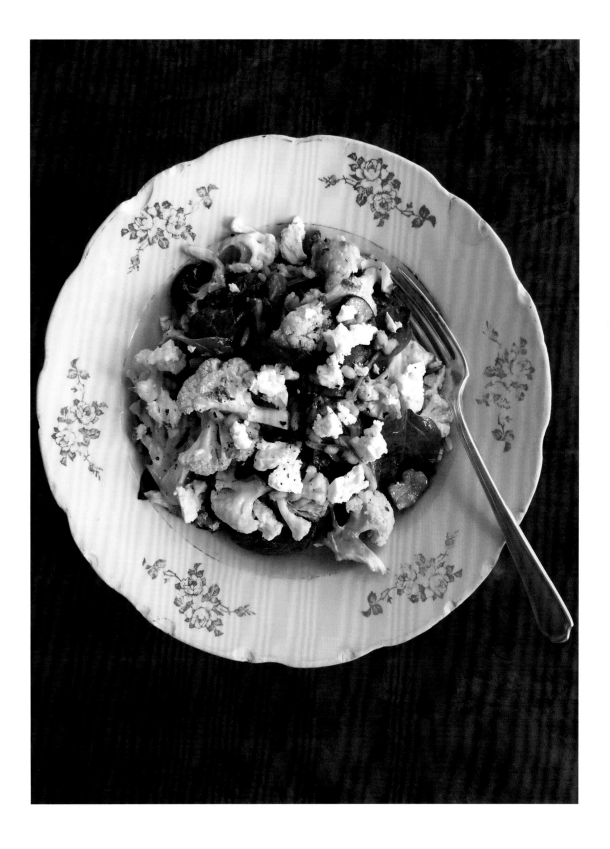

Baby Root Vegetables with Balsamic and Chèvre

 4–6   PREP: 15 min   COOKING TIME: 30 min   GF

INGREDIENTS:

200ml **balsamic vinegar**

2 tbsp **honey**

several sprigs of **rosemary**

1kg mix of **baby root vegetables,** washed

olive oil

salt and **pepper**

150g (5oz) **chèvre** or **other soft white cheese**

Preheat the oven to 200°C on fan grill.

Combine the balsamic, honey and rosemary in a small saucepan over a low heat and let it gently reduce by half, which will take about 10 minutes. Be especially careful not to let it burn. Once it has reduced, take off the heat and allow it to cool.

In the meantime, bring a large saucepan of salted water to the boil. Quickly blanch the vegetables in batches according to variety; turnips and beetroot will need a little longer than baby carrots, which will need barely a minute. Baby leeks won't need long either. You want to retain some crunch. Drain and refresh the vegetables under cold water, drain again then spread them out on an oiled baking tray.

Roast the vegetables until they are caramelised and a little crisp on the outside, about 20 minutes. Remove from the oven, and set aside to cool. Remove the rosemary sprigs and transfer the cooled vegetables to a large bowl, pour the balsamic mixture over them and toss well to coat.

To serve, arrange the vegetables on a plate, crumble the chèvre on top.

Sam: You can use pretty much any sort of root vegetable. Baby turnips, swedes, beetroot, leeks, fennel bulbs and baby carrots (which now come in a whole spectrum of colours) are all pretty decent options. And while chèvre can be a little strong for some people, a nice creamy feta or even some ricotta will work well as an alternative.

Karen: Not only does the fragrant herb rosemary add a delicious x-factor to this recipe, it also contains substances that are useful for stimulating the immune system, increasing circulation, and improving digestion.

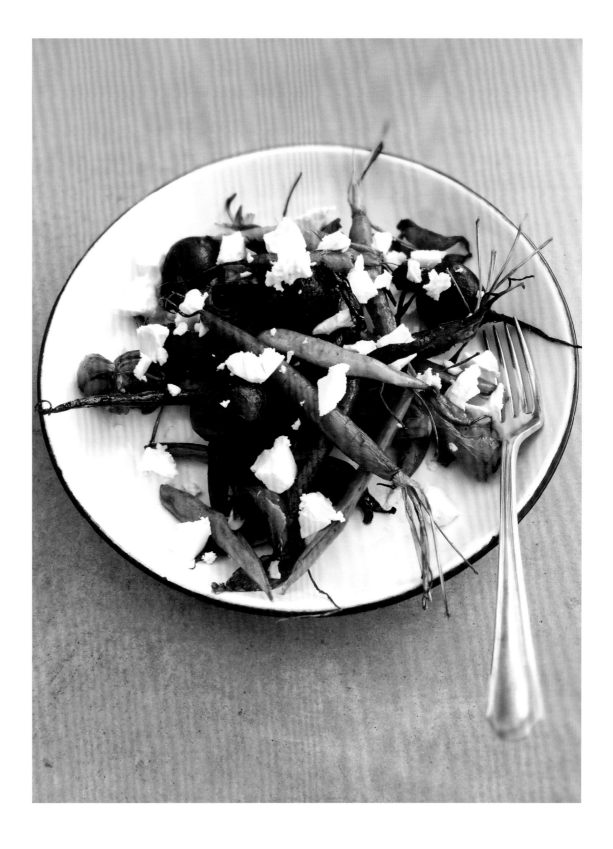

New Potatoes with Feta, Beans, Turmeric and Parsley

4–6   PREP: 10 min   COOKING TIME: 10 min   GF

INGREDIENTS:

900g (32oz) **new potatoes**, scrubbed

200g (7oz) **long green beans**, ends removed

olive oil

2 tsp ground **turmeric**

1 tbsp **cumin seeds**, toasted

salt and **pepper**

small handful of **parsley**, roughly chopped

150g (5oz) **feta**

Halve the spuds if necessary, then boil in plenty of salted water until they are tender. Drain and transfer to a large bowl.

Blanch the beans in boiling water for about 1 minute – you want them to retain their fresh crunch so take care not to overcook them. Run under cold water to cool them down, then drain and add to the potatoes. Add 1–2 tablespoons olive oil, followed by all the remaining ingredients except for the feta. Toss everything together to combine.

Taste and season accordingly, then transfer to a serving platter or dish. Scatter the feta over the top and serve.

Sam: This is an astoundingly simple recipe, which makes a delicious, substantial meal on its own. Turmeric is a bit of a hero in this case (I love the stuff). You can use ricotta or paneer instead of feta, although I think the feta adds a nice creamy sharpness. Heat leftovers of this up in a pan so that the cheese melts and goes everywhere.

Karen: As well as tasting great, turmeric is a potent anti-inflammatory and antioxidant. It is also good for improving cognitive function and blood sugar balance. Enjoy this recipe for its taste and wonderful health benefits.

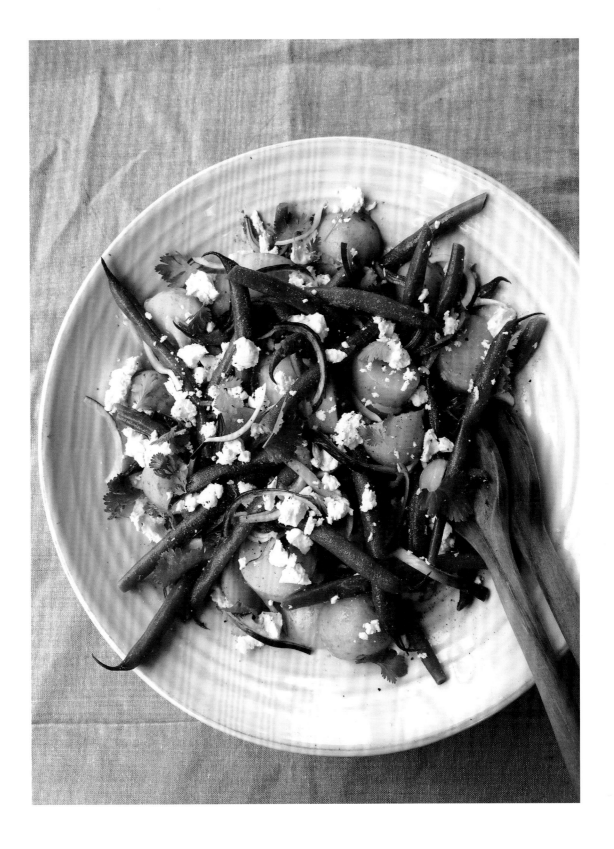

Common side effects of hormone therapy

HOW TO MINIMISE THE SYMPTOMS

'I started taking Tamoxifen and had a real problem with weight gain and hot flushes. Thankfully I have an excellent GP, and she suggested many practical things that have helped.' – Judy

'The thing I noticed about hormone therapy was how dry I felt, my skin, my hair and internally. I've changed the products I use, and I'm fussier now about my diet.' – Sarah

Many people are on hormone therapy following a cancer diagnosis. Hormone therapy, for people with cancers that are hormone sensitive or hormone dependent, is the use of medicines to block the effects of hormones. Some people find they have little or no symptoms; a number of men with prostate cancer will experience symptoms that are discussed later in the chapter while some women experience symptoms that are similar to going through menopause.

To find out more, I spoke to Dr. Janice Brown, a general practitioner and clinical director at Auckland University, who specialises in women's health, and in particular menopause. Dr Brown is also on the education committee for the Australasian Menopause Board. We met on a summer's day and the following pages reflect our discussion on solutions for some of the common symptoms.

HOT FLUSHES AND NIGHT SWEATS

Women describe having a hot flush as heat that floods their whole body, which can also make them red and sweaty. Night sweats can keep women awake. While both of these symptoms can be minor in some cases they are very distressing and can have a negative impact on quality of life. In terms of a solution, Dr Brown says it very much depends on the individual woman.

'It's best to see a health professional, like myself, who has expertise in the area. SNRI and SSRI anti-depressants can be used to treat hot flushes and night sweats, and in the right doses they can reduce symptoms by 60–70 per cent on average. Check with your doctor to ensure there are no adverse drug reactions, however.'

Small lifestyle changes can also help:

- Regular exercise, improved diet, stopping smoking and reducing alcohol and caffeine intake will improve overall health and can make symptoms easier to tolerate.

- Dressing in layers is practical.

- Avoid spicy food.

- At night time, use bed covers that are easy to remove.

- Place a fan near you that you can turn on as needed.

- Some people find hypnosis to be helpful.

At all costs avoid compounded bioidentical hormonal preparations. They are not recommended due to major concerns about their safety and efficacy. While there are a number of herbal products touted as providing relief from menopausal symptoms check with a health professional to see if they have been shown in clinical studies to be safe and effective, ie don't necessarily believe the marketing hype on the package. Just because they claim to be 'natural' doesn't mean they will be helpful – and in some cases, they may be harmful.

SLEEP PROBLEMS

Again, Dr Brown recommends talking to your doctor if you are having trouble sleeping.

'A doctor will do a full assessment to see what is stopping a person from sleeping.

Are they having trouble falling asleep or are they waking up? Are they hot and sweaty when they wake up? If so, then it might be the hot flushes or night sweats waking them. But sleeping problems could be caused by depression, which is very common, and one of the first things depression can affect is sleep. Or it could be some of the medication a person is on that is making sleep difficult.

'If there is no medical or drug reason for them not sleeping then I would look at sleep hygiene. It's important in this case to have a routine in the evening. No screens an hour before bed. TV or reading on a Kindle is OK, but not a tablet or phone. It's important to do the same thing every night until your body gets into the routine of sleeping again.'

MOOD CHANGES

Any changes in mood could be to do with the side effects of hormone treatment, but there may be other reasons.

'A major medical diagnosis, chemo, radiotherapy and exhaustion – these are all reasons why someone might be moody. A medical professional can assess you,

to see if it is the drugs you are on, but if it's not that, it might be useful for you to see a psychologist; not so much for counselling, but for learning some good techniques, such as cognitive behaviour therapy or mindfulness, so you learn good ways to manage how you are feeling.

'But you may be clinically depressed, in which case there is a questionnaire for you to fill in which can often trigger your thoughts on the subject and that can be very helpful. PHQ9 self-assessments can be found online.

'The most important thing is to be honest when doing these questionnaires. It won't be seen by anyone else except you and your health professional. It uses the numbers 1, 2, 3 and 4 as a rating, so you can't be in the middle. And because it has nine questions it is called the PHQ9.'

WEIGHT GAIN

Many women struggle with a menopausal type of weight gain when they are on hormone therapy, mostly tending to put on weight around the midriff.

'This kind of weight gain is annoying for people, especially if they have had a slim waist before. I recommend that they see a dietician if it is problematic. And look to reduce processed carbohydrates and eat a healthy well-balanced diet. What most women don't realise is that after menopause,

and when on hormonal treatments, they probably need a third less food than what they previously needed. So it's good to look at what they're eating if they are putting on weight and storing it around their middle. It may be that now they need to reduce the size of their portions.

'Exercise is good because it makes your metabolism work more efficiently. Walking is easy to do, and it's not just about the calories you burn, but that it makes your system more efficient for the next 24 hours. There is a lot of evidence now about the importance of moving. So get out there and walk, go swimming, play tennis, go cycling – whatever appeals. If you are bedridden, then start doing things with your arms. Being immobile is not good, so think about how you can get moving. A lot of people who have surgery don't mobilise – but it makes a huge difference to their recovery and mental health if they can do some exercise.

'Being on hormone treatment is a chemical menopause for women to a certain degree. This can involve muscle wasting very quickly, and bone loss, too, if they are not careful. Women on hormone therapy need to get weight bearing exercise going. So exercise not just for your weight, but for your bones, strength and your mental health.

'Women on hormone treatment can also be at a higher risk of osteoporosis, so it's good to build up muscle strength in the arms, legs and in your core area, which you can strengthen by walking and moving around. Or get some weights, even a couple of spaghetti cans can work well. You don't have to go out and spend a lot of money. There is a lot of good evidence that women who exercise have a much better cancer prognosis.'

If you are experiencing weight gain and wish to make changes to your diet, the recipes in the salad and soups section of this book will be of great interest.

DRYNESS

Dry skin and hair is very common among people on hormone therapy. Some also encounter dry mouths, while vaginal dryness can be a huge problem for women, although this particular symptom is often not talked about.

'The best thing you can do for dry hair and skin is to eat fresh fruit and vegetables, so you are getting as many minerals as possible into your body. Dryness is a problem for women after menopause per se, so I think that whoever comes up with a solution will end up being very wealthy!

'Eat lots of salmon which is high in fish oils; flaxseed is also particularly good for combating dryness. I'm not really into supplements as I'm not sure how active the ingredients are once they are in the capsules and have sat on the supermarket shelf for weeks before being bought so I'd encourage people to get the nutrients they need from the food they eat.

'From a moisturising point of view, I recommend non-scented, thick and greasy creams because your skin can become more sensitive, eg Cetomacrogol cream which is available by prescription. For a dry mouth, chewing gum or sucking mints can stimulate saliva. Or ask your doctor to prescribe an oral lubricant.'

Vaginal dryness affects many women on hormone therapy. Here are some practical tips that may help:

- Minimise irritation by wearing pure cotton underwear (or other natural fibres).

- Don't wear underwear in bed.

- Use low-allergenic washing products.

- Don't use feminine hygiene sprays or douche.

- Use unscented pads, tampons and toilet paper.

- Avoid shaving or waxing the genital area.

Make up a cool wash or compress to help itching and mild discomfort by dissolving half a teaspoon of bicarbonate of soda in 1 litre of water. Apply gently with a cloth a few times a day.

Being sexually active may improve your symptoms as sexual activity improves blood flow and helps maintain healthy tissue. Consider using a water or silicone-based vaginal lubricant or moisturiser to reduce friction and make intercourse more comfortable.

Quit smoking. There are many reasons for doing so but smoking actually decreases blood flow to the genital area, directly affecting vaginal cells.

Vitamin E, taken orally or applied as an ointment, can reduce symptoms.

For ongoing troublesome symptoms, talk to your oncologist about the possibility of using a topical vaginal hormonal preparation, which can be very effective. There is also emerging interest in CO2 laser therapy, which in basic terms, 'remodels' the vagina with healthier tissue – but studies are still being done in this area, so you are best to talk to your doctor.

ESPECIALLY FOR MEN
While the previous information relates to women taking hormone therapy, men who are on hormone therapy for prostate cancer

may also experience symptoms to a greater or lesser extent. Symptoms can include:

- a lowered libido

- erectile dysfunction

- loss of bone density, muscle mass and physical strength

- weight gain

- hot flushes

- mood swings

- fatigue

Much of the advice offered to women is also applicable to men, especially a well-balanced diet and exercise. This can help manage symptoms, including extreme tiredness. Regular resistance exercise such as fast walking, swimming and exercising with small weights may help to reduce muscle loss and keep muscles and bones strong.

However, for obvious reasons the sexual side effects of hormone therapy for prostate cancer can be the most difficult to deal with. Erectile dysfunction drugs usually do not work for men who are experiencing a lack of sexual desire. In this case it would pay to seek professional help, particularly to establish if depression may be the cause. It's recommended to undertake a quick questionnaire to rule this out as depression is very common among people going through cancer treatments.

IN SUMMARY

Men and women may feel uncomfortable talking to their health professional about some of the symptoms, but it really is worth talking to someone who specialises in this area to find out what can be done to help.

Your cancer specialists will be used to talking about these symptoms so do speak out if they are bothering you. Don't suffer in silence, get the help you need.

Dealing with pain and discomfort

'Recovering from surgery was a lot less painful than I had anticipated, but I must admit I felt a bit sore for some time.' — Jeremy

'While the pain medication seemed to work well, I also found complementary treatments helped me while I was recovering from surgery and the cancer treatments.' — Alice

Cancer patients often have to deal with pain after surgery, and sometimes during treatment, too. Pain is a symptom that decreases the quality of life and which can also hinder the recovery process. It should not be ignored. Any pain or discomfort you may experience should be discussed with a health professional as there is a good chance that it can be controlled. Take any medication that's been specifically prescribed to best keep on top of any pain. Don't be tempted to skip a dose, as it may not then be as effective. Here are some tips that may further help the situation.

Heat packs: hot water bottles or wheat bags that can be warmed in the microwave are a good way to apply heat to a specific part of the body so you can target pain relief where it is most needed. An ice or gel pack can be used as a cold compress to alleviate the pain of minor injuries. These can be purchased at most local pharmacies.

BREATHING

It's only natural to want to breathe shallowly when you are in pain, but deep, gentle breathing from your diaphragm can actually help with any pain you are experiencing.

Put yourself in a relaxed, reclining position, then either shut your eyes or look straight ahead. Gently place your hand on your belly and begin a long, slow breath, breathing through your nostrils. Let the breath go down to your diaphragm so you can feel it pushing against your hand. Don't hold your breath; just pause and then exhale. Imagine, if you like, a balloon in your belly inflating and deflating as you do this. Then inhale again, long and slow, and repeat the process until you feel the pain lessen.

If you start to feel dizzy or faint, return to your normal breathing pattern for a while, slow down your exhalations, or lengthen the natural pause between your inhale and your exhale.

As well as helping to manage physical pain, breathing from your diaphragm can reduce anxiety, depression, and stress by turning your body off from 'fight or flight' mode. It also enhances the immune system, improves lymphatic flow, cardiovascular health and blood chemistry.

EXERCISE AND PHYSIOTHERAPY

I invited Lou James, the physiotherapist who founded the PINC & STEEL Cancer Rehabilitation Trust to discuss the role of exercise in relieving pain.

'In my profession we often deal with pain, which can cause a whole lot of worry and also functional problems. It's important not to put up with pain, but to seek help. Any of the usual cancer treatments can cause pain. In cancer surgery, you can get pain if they cut nerves. Chemotherapy can cause pain through the nerves and the toxicity of the drugs. Then there's lymphoedema, which can cause pain. Myopathy (a disease of muscle tissue) can also cause pain. So many things can cause pain, but there are also a lot of ways to relieve it.

'Sometimes things become painful when you are not moving properly. Scar tissue can be painful if it adheres, so manual physiotherapy or mobilisations are needed. If you can free up something that is painful and stiff, you can often reduce pain.'

Lou advises people to talk to their oncologist if they are experiencing pain as a result of treatment as it can sometimes be changed if it is causing these distressing symptoms.

'Oncologists want to know if there are any adverse reactions, but people can be very reluctant to say if they are having problems. They might worry that their treatment will be suspended, but there are a lot of different chemotherapy drugs these days. People need to speak up and just be honest about any symptoms they may have.

'If you don't do anything about pain, it can sometimes turn into chronic pain, but if you address things early you can stop it from developing into a bigger problem. For example, when women have surgery on their breast, around their shoulders, head or neck, it often has a significant implication on the way they move their arms, which can lead to long-term problems unless it gets sorted. A lot of cancer rehabilitation physiotherapy is often movement-based. We look at how your body is moving and functioning, and we will work with you to make sure you improve your function.'

For some people it might not be possible to return to their old selves 100% after surgery, but there are still many benefits to be gained from seeking help from a physiotherapist regarding exercises to improve function.

'We see a lot of people with cancers that impact on bowel, bladder, and sexual function. And often people don't want to talk about these things. They think, "This is just my lot, I've had surgery and it's probably going to be like this from now on." But often this is not the case. If you can be assessed by someone who is a trained cancer rehabilitation physiotherapist, someone who understands all the mechanics, you can often get a lot of control and strength back. My biggest worry is that so many people end up having symptoms which they put up with for life, because they didn't know about the support on offer to which their doctor could have referred them.

'Everyone focuses on the cancer, but when the cancer is gone people still want to be able to function as best they can, and not to be in pain. If they get seen early we can work on things that strengthen and help all areas recover, rather than not doing anything. It is obvious that if people are proactive and get support with movement during their treatments, they will get through the treatments and the other side better.'

COMPLEMENTARY THERAPIES

Some people find complementary therapies help with pain, but note that they don't work for everyone. If you decide to use a complementary therapy, you should always talk to your health professional first and be aware that complementary therapies should not replace any treatments prescribed by your doctor.

Some of the many different treatments and therapies available include massage, acupuncture, meditation, TENS and hypnosis.

Massage

Massage may be helpful in reducing tension and pain, improving blood flow, and encouraging relaxation. Massage therapists usually apply pressure with their hands, but they can also use their forearms, elbows, or feet. You can choose from many different types of massage: some gentle, some very active and intense. When done properly, massage is considered safe. But always consult your doctor first, particularly if:

- you have open wounds, bruises, or areas of weak skin

- you have a bleeding disorder, have low blood platelet counts, or are taking a blood thinner medicine

- you have a blood clot in a vein.

Acupuncture

Practised for centuries, acupuncture is a form of traditional Chinese medicine which some cancer patients find helpful for relieving pain. Acupuncture is based on the theory that chi (energy) flows through and around your body. Practitioners believe that illness or pain occurs when something blocks or unbalances your chi, so this treatment is a way to unblock or influence chi and help it flow back into balance.

Acupuncture involves the practitioner putting very thin needles into your skin at certain points on your body to influence the energy flow. Sometimes heat, pressure, or mild electrical current is used along with needles. While treatment can vary, in most cases it lasts for 15 minutes to an hour. You may be invited to make several visits to complete your treatment. And while most people find that it doesn't hurt, some report feeling slight pressure when a needle goes in and the area around it may tingle or itch.

Meditation

Some people find mindful meditation helpful in reducing ongoing pain. While it is not likely to be a cure-all for every pain, many cancer patients have reported that it can bring relief.

There is no right or wrong way to meditate and there are many books and recordings that will help you get started. Typically they recommend finding a quiet, dark room to meditate in, starting with ten-minute blocks.

Transcutaneous electrical nerve stimulation (TENS or TNS)

TENS devices are used as a non-invasive nerve stimulation intended to reduce both acute and chronic pain. While studies around its success in reducing pain are conflicting, it is clear that some people benefit from using these devices.

A TENS unit is usually connected to the skin using two or more electrodes and is typically battery-operated to modulate pulse frequency and intensity.

Hypnosis

Hypnosis is a successful way of managing pain for some people. More often it helps the person manage pain by redirecting their attention away from the sensation of pain. Sessions may vary in length, but are generally somewhere between 10 and 20 minutes. A session will often begin with a focus on your breathing to help you relax. Then the hypnotist will most likely direct you to imagine a pleasant place which you describe in detail, such as being on the beach on a warm sunny day. The idea behind it is that while you will feel the same sensation of pain, you'll be in much less distress about it because you will also be experiencing the pleasure of being in a special place.

In summary, never ignore any pain you might be experiencing. Always talk to your doctor about it, especially if you wish to seek other ways as discussed above to manage it.

The symptoms you don't want to talk about

'It's the things that people don't see that are the hardest. They are not things you want to share with other people as they are so personal and private.'
— Mairi

'The treatments and their symptoms are not forever – even though it seems that way some days. There are more people out there going through this than you think. You can get through this.' — Jessica

There can be a number of symptoms from cancer treatments that you may feel embarrassed or uncomfortable talking about. Here are some practical tips for combating some of these symptoms.

MOUTH ULCERS

It's not uncommon to develop mouth ulcers when undergoing chemotherapy. However, OraSoothe has been developed by health professionals to help ease the pain and support the healing of oral wounds and lesions. It provides fast pain relief without a numbing sensation, it helps prevent microbial contamination, and it promotes optimal healing.

You might like to try making an easy home-made mouthwash by mixing together 1 teaspoon of salt and 1 teaspoon of sodium bicarbonate in 200ml of warm water. If you find it helps, make a fresh batch each day and use to rinse out your mouth after each main meal.

DIARRHOEA

Experiencing diarrhoea when undergoing cancer treatment is very common. However, if it is significant or persistent, you should seek prompt medical attention as there are effective anti-diarrhoea medications (ie loperamide) available; your health professional may also need to test a sample to exclude the possibility of infection. In the meantime, it's recommended that you:

- Avoid certain foods including milk, yoghurt, dairy desserts and ice-cream as you may have a temporary lactose intolerance. When you no longer have diarrhoea, you can gradually reintroduce dairy products back into your diet. Other foods to avoid during this time are greasy, high fibre or sugary foods. And no caffeine.

Keep hydrated by ensuring that you drink plenty of fluids, taking small, frequent sips if necessary rather than large quantities at any time. Water is, of course, very important but clear thin broths or soups are also good. Minimise your electrolyte losses with diluted non-caffeinated sports drinks and try ice blocks, and lemonade for a refreshing way to keep up your fluids. Rehydration formulations are available from your pharmacy.

- Activated charcoal can be used in the short term to treat diarrhoea. It's an inexpensive remedy that is simple to take, especially in capsule form, and which dates back thousands of years to the time of the ancient Egyptians. Similar to common charcoal, the activated variety is made especially for use as a medicine by heating it in the presence of a gas that causes the charcoal to develop lots of internal spaces or pores that help the substance trap chemicals. Talk to your doctor about the suitability of taking activated charcoal, and note that it should not be used for children under three years of age.

- Surprisingly, grated apples, mixed with honey and left in a bowl until they turn brown, make an effective remedy for diarrhoea. This is because apples create a soluble fibre known as pectin which has a regulating effect on the speed of digestion.

Check out the recipes for various teas and the chapter on soups where you'll find delicious ideas that will help if you are experiencing diarrhoea.

CONSTIPATION

Certain drugs, especially morphine, can cause problematic constipation. Here are some ideas to help:

Increase the amount of fibre in your diet, especially by eating more fruit and vegetables. All of the following contain good amounts of fibre: apricots, berries, beans, broccoli, plums, pears, oranges, figs and kiwifruit.

- Prunes are one of the oldest home remedies for constipation. High in fibre, prunes also contain a compound called dihydroxy phenyl isatin, which kick starts the colon into action.

- Black licorice can have a laxative effect.

- Flaxseed oil, another simple home remedy for constipation, is high in fibre and contains heart-healthy omega-3 fats. Ideally take one tablespoon two or three times a day, adding it to your morning cereal or smoothie.

- Sip water steadily during the day so it can be absorbed into your body. Herbal teas or a simple cup of hot water with lemon juice taken regularly will also help.

- Dandelion tea can have a mildly laxative effect if taken three times per day. It's also easy to make: simply steep one teaspoon of the dried root in one cup of boiling water.

- Get moving! Exercise will help so aim for regular short walks if you can.

If none of the above works for you, ask your doctor to recommend an appropriate laxative.

The chapter on salads contain various ingredients that will help alleviate constipation as will the following recipes:

- Gratin of Pumpkin, Leek, Lentils and Hazelnuts, page 92

- Yam, Silverbeet and Feta Galettes, page 94

- Sam's Spanakopita with Walnuts, Pine Nuts, Silverbeet and Mint, page 96

- Spring Risotto of Asparagus, Broad Beans, Lemon & Feta, page 102

- Curry of Pumpkin, Snake Beans, Cashews and Curry Leaves, page 112

- Wild Rice, Salmon, Edamame and Pickled Ginger, page 122

REFLUX

Some cancer patients will struggle with reflux issues, which can be helped by using either over-the-counter or prescription medications. However, also consider the following tips to help alleviate this problem:

- Reflux tends to be worse at night when you are lying down. Try elevating your head by around 10cm if possible and avoid trying to sleep for a couple of hours after eating.

- Eat slowly and take time to chew your food, which will allow your stomach enough time to digest without pumping out excess acid.

- Avoid foods high in acid, such as tomatoes or citrus fruits, and foods that are spicy.

- Add some raw, unfiltered apple cider vinegar to your drinking water as it is thought that this home remedy can help balance your stomach pH by neutralising stomach acid.

- Certain fruits, particularly bananas, contain natural antacids that can act as a buffer against acid reflux. Apples can also be known to bring some relief so snack on one a couple of hours before bedtime. Interestingly, for this condition, sweet apples are thought to be better than sour varieties.

- As well as helping with symptoms of nausea, ginger is also good at combating reflux.

- Some people find snacking on a few almonds after a meal can relieve reflux.

- Surprisingly mustard, an alkalising food full of minerals, can be helpful. Consuming half a teaspoon of commercial mustard straight from the jar (just whatever flavour you enjoy) will help neutralise the acid that may come creeping up your throat and therefore counteract the pain of acid reflux.

- Many people already enjoy a cup of chamomile tea before bedtime as not only does it aid sleep but it also helps reduce inflammation in your stomach and possibly balances out the acidity levels as well.

Your doctor will be able to provide you with effective anti-reflux medications if reflux is occurring despite dietary manipulation.

LYMPHOEDEMA

Lymphoedema can occur following breast cancer surgery and/or radiotherapy. It is the accumulation of lymphatic fluid in an area of the body due of the removal of lymph nodes or the obstruction of lymphatic vessels. It can develop in the arm, on the same side as the treated armpit, or in the remaining breast tissue left on the chest after mastectomy or after breast-conserving surgery. It usually develops gradually and can appear long after treatment. Causing a feeling of swelling, tightness, discomfort and pain, it can't be cured but there are some things you can do to manage it such as:

Keep your skin hydrated. Dry skin can lead to cracked skin which in turn could provide an entry for bacteria that increases the risk of infection. Avoid sunburn or any form of burn on the affected area, also hot baths or saunas, and insect bites.

Take preventative measures such as wearing gloves when gardening and doing dishes. Do not allow the affected arm to be used when having your blood pressure taken, or an injection or blood test. Avoid heavy lifting, but gentle exercise such as walking and swimming is especially effective. Consult your doctor before a long haul flight about the need to wear a compression sleeve. And if you think you have an infection in your arm, see your doctor immediately.

Keeping active through exercise and also maintaining a healthy BMI will help manage the symptoms of lymphoedema.

During the course of my research I met with Sinda to discuss the ongoing implications of lymphoedema that occurred after her cancer diagnosis.

'Lymphoedema has been the thing I have struggled with the most. I'm a keen swimmer, but for some time I was scared to swim. I was worried about making my lymphoedema worse, yet I knew jolly well from everything I'd read that I should be exercising. But the hydrostatic pressure of water is actually really good and I've gone on to do ocean swims, raising money for charity.

'Another thing I struggled with was shopping for new clothes. Having to wear that special skin-coloured sleeve made me anxious because I didn't want anyone to notice it. And even though it is skin coloured, I just couldn't bear it because I was sure everyone was looking at me, I had a real thing about it. You wear a sleeveless dress, and you can see it. So I started buying all these baggy long-sleeved shirts, and it took me a long time to not worry about it.

'It was hard to come to terms with the fact that once you've got it, you've got it. I'll have to contend with lymphoedema for life; I didn't realise that to begin with. Every time I go on a flight, I have to be careful. Every time I go swimming in seas where there is coral I have to be careful not to graze my arm or cut my hand and get an infection that way. And I am especially mindful about insect bites.'

Sinda eventually found that joining a lymphoedema network and getting to hear other people's stories and tips was very helpful. And while she can't change having lymphoedema, there are things she can do to help herself, such as maintaining her BMI and doing lots of exercise, along with looking after her skin and taking preventative measures to stop cuts, bites and burns. Various support networks can be found online, or you can ask your doctor.

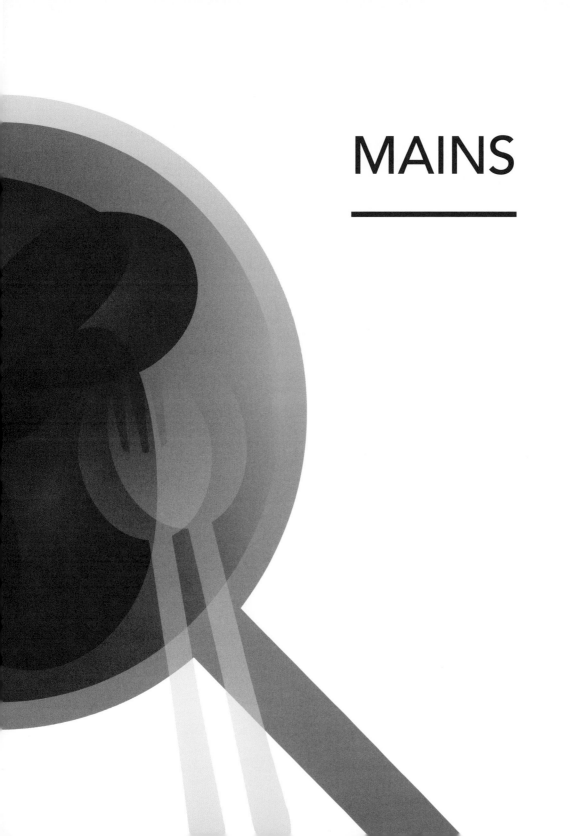

MAINS

Gratin of Pumpkin, Leek, Lentils and Hazelnuts

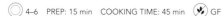 4–6   PREP: 15 min   COOKING TIME: 45 min   GF

INGREDIENTS:

2kg (70oz) **crown** or **butternut pumpkin**, peeled, deseeded and diced into 2–3cm chunks

olive oil

1 tbsp **butter**

1 **leek**, thoroughly washed and finely sliced

several sprigs of **rosemary** and **thyme leaves** removed from stems

1 tsp **Dijon mustard**

½ cup (125ml) **dry white wine**

¼ cup (62.5ml) **cream**

400g (14oz) **Puy lentils**, cooked and drained

2–3 tablespoons grated **parmesan**

¼ cup (37.5g/1.3oz) **hazelnuts**, toasted and roughly chopped

Preheat the oven to 180°C. Place the pumpkin in a roasting tray, toss with a little olive oil and salt and pepper and roast for 20–25 minutes until tender.

In the meantime, in a pan over a medium heat, add the butter and allow to bubble up before adding the leek and fresh herbs. Cook gently for 5–10 minutes until the leek is soft and translucent. Add the mustard and fry for 1 minute, then add the white wine and allow to it to reduce a little. Follow with the cream and let it bubble up and cook for a minute or two. Finally, add the cooked lentils, stir and take off the heat.

Gently fold the cooked pumpkin into the leek and lentil mixture. Taste and season accordingly, then transfer the mixture to a ceramic baking dish or oven-proof pan. Sprinkle the grated parmesan over the top to cover the mixture. Pop in the oven and let the parmesan melt into the pumpkin mixture, then remove from the oven and scatter over the hazelnuts. Serve immediately.

Sam: Fresh local hazelnuts will always put imported ones to shame. Gently toast them in the oven before eating; this will enhance the flavour significantly. Swap ingredients as you see fit – kumara or yams are good replacements for pumpkin, as are toasted walnuts in lieu of hazelnuts. This dish is a delight on its own, or for those with a good appetite serve it as a substantial side dish.

Karen: Lentils are packed with nutrition and are a great source of fibre, iron, protein, Vitamins B1 and B6, zinc and potassium. This is small but mighty food to include in your diet.

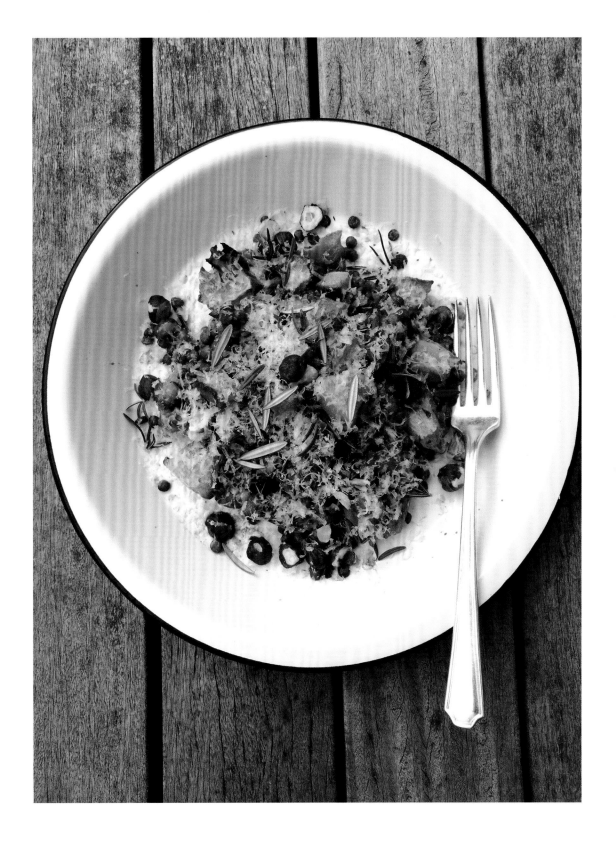

Yam, Silverbeet and Feta Galettes

4–6   PREP: 10 min   COOKING TIME: 35-45 min

INGREDIENTS:

800g (28oz) **yams**

olive oil

salt and **pepper**

12 sprigs of **rosemary**

1 bunch **silverbeet**

100g (3.5oz) **feta**

1 **egg**, lightly beaten

1 tsp **pomegranate molasses** (optional)

salt and **pepper**

500g (17.5oz) **savoury shortcrust pastry**

Preheat the oven to 180°C. Scrub the yams, slice them up into 1cm pieces and place in a roasting tray with a little olive oil, salt and pepper and a bit of the rosemary. Roast until tender but not too soft. You don't want them turning to mush. Set aside to cool.

Wash the silverbeet, wring out the moisture, trim off the stalks and chop roughly. Crumble the feta into a large bowl. Add the silverbeet and the beaten egg and mix well with your hands so that everything is combined. Add the pomegranate molasses and fold in the yams. Taste the mixture and season accordingly.

Lay the pastry out on a floured surface. Using a small plate (about 180cm diameter is good), cut out rounds of pastry. Spread fist-sized blobs of the yam and silverbeet mixture in the centre, leaving a 2cm gap around the edge, then fold the edges over, pleating as you go, so that you end up with an open-topped pie. Carefully place the galettes on a lined tray and bake for a further 15–20 minutes until the pastry is all lovely and golden. Serve with a simple salad on the side.

Sam: This recipe is more of a guideline, so chop and change filling ingredients as you see fit. Bear in mind that you don't want the filling to be too wet or the pastry will be soggy on the bottom. Pomegranate molasses, if you like the idea, will add a sweet-sour edge.

Karen: Silverbeet is a wonder food. As well as being a good source of iron, potassium and manganese, it has Vitamins A, C, E and K.

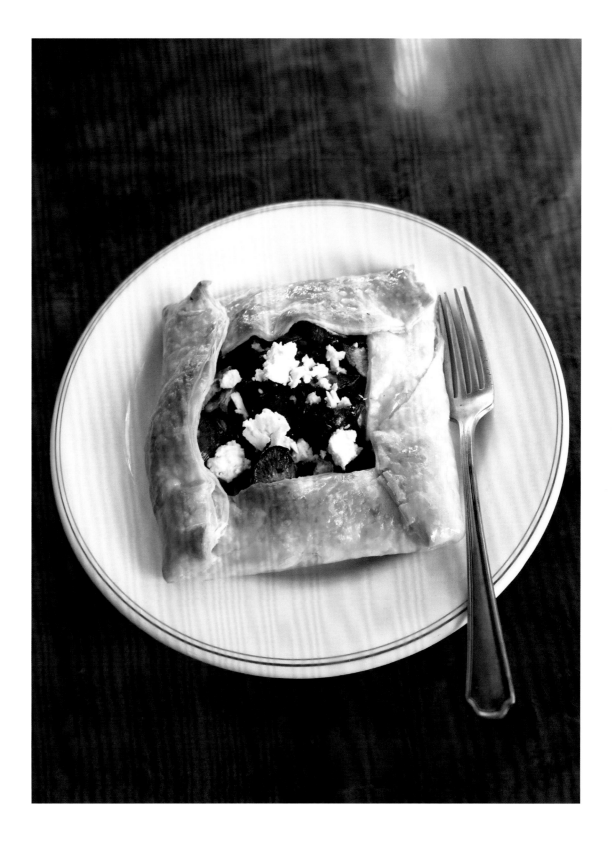

Sam's Spanakopita with Walnuts, Pine Nuts, Silverbeet and Mint

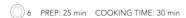 6   PREP: 25 min   COOKING TIME: 30 min

INGREDIENTS:

olive oil

100g (3.5oz) **butter**, melted

1 **onion**, finely chopped

1 **fennel bulb**, cored and finely sliced, fronds reserved and chopped

1 large bunch of **silverbeet**, washed

250g (8.8oz) **filo pastry**

zest of 2 **lemons**

100g (1.7oz) **feta**, crumbled

50g (3.5oz) **cheddar**, grated

100g **cottage cheese** or **ricotta**

½ tsp freshly grated **nutmeg**

2 **eggs**, lightly beaten

½ cup (62.5g/2.2oz) **walnuts**, toasted and roughly chopped

¼ cup (35g/1.2oz) **pine nuts**, toasted

large handful of **mint leaves**, chopped

large handful of **flat-leaf parsley**, stalks included, chopped

handful of **rocket**

salt and **black pepper**

Preheat the oven to 180°C. In a large saucepan over a medium heat add a little olive oil and a tablespoon of the butter and let it bubble and foam up. Add the onion and sliced fennel bulb and cook gently for 5 minutes or so until translucent.

Separate the silverbeet stalks from the leaves. Chop the stalks finely and add them the onion mix. Cook for another couple of minutes until the stalks have softened, then slice up the leaves and add to the mix until they are slightly wilted. Remove from the heat and set aside to cool. In the meantime, grease a roasting tray with some of the melted butter and line with 4 layers of filo pastry, ensuring a bit of overlap over the sides, brushing each sheet with melted butter in between.

Add the lemon zest, feta, cheddar, cottage cheese or ricotta, grated nutmeg and beaten egg to the cooled silverbeet mixture and mix in well so that everything is combined. Fold in the walnuts, pine nuts, mint, parsley, rocket and reserved fennel fronds. Taste and season accordingly with lots of salt and freshly ground black pepper.

Spread the mixture over the top of the filo pastry in the tin, smooth off, and then layer with some more filo, brushing each sheet with butter as you go. Trim and pinch the edges together, brush the top with a little more butter, then bake for 25–30 minutes until the pastry is lovely and golden. Allow to cool a little before serving.

Sam: You will find wonderful variations of this recipe all around the Eastern Mediterranean, but the common thread between them all is that nobody ever skimps on the herbs.

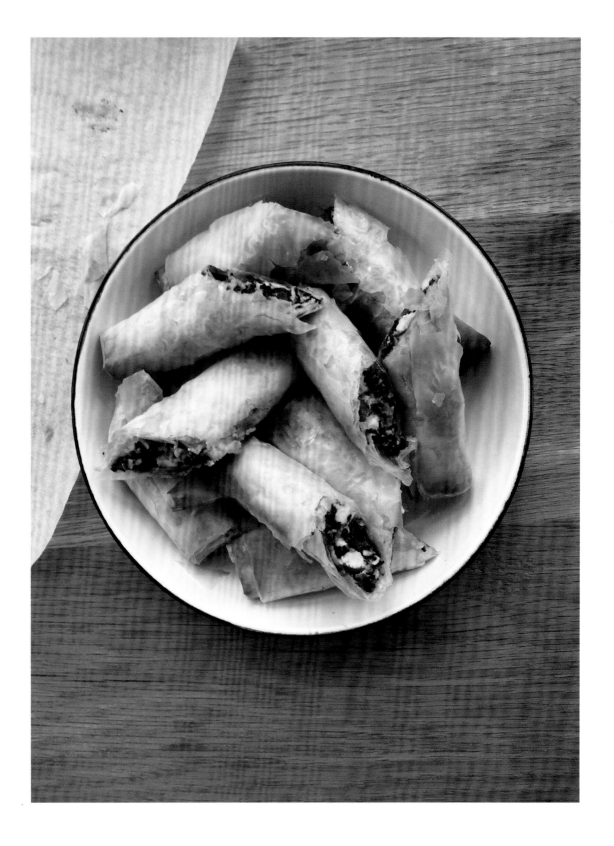

Kumara, Red Onion and Coriander Fritters

4–6   PREP: 10 min   COOKING TIME: 30 min   GF

INGREDIENTS:

2 large **kumara**, scrubbed and cut into chunks

1 **red onion**, peeled and sliced into thin wedges

olive oil

salt and **pepper**

1 tsp **cumin seeds**

1 tbsp grated **parmesan**

handful of **coriander**, finely chopped (stalks included)

2 **eggs**, lightly beaten

50g (1.7oz) **butter**, for frying

Preheat the oven to 180°C.

Toss the kumara and red onion with a bit of olive oil in a roasting dish. Season with salt and pepper, then bake for 20 minutes or so until the kumara is soft and the onion is nicely caramelised. Remove and allow to cool. Transfer the cooled kumara and onion to a mixing bowl and mash everything up a bit. Add the cumin, parmesan and chopped coriander, and mix well. Fold in the beaten egg and season.

Add the butter and a little olive oil to a frying pan over a moderate heat. Add a little more olive oil and a bit of butter between batches as necessary and fry dollops of the mixture gently for several minutes on each side until golden brown. Pop the cooked fritters on top of a paper towel to drain off excess oil while you cook the rest.

Serve immediately, while they are still warm.

Sam: I'm not a fan of using flour in fritters as I think it makes them a bit stodgy. The kumara and egg act well enough as a binder. If chilli is your thing, throw some in. You may want to add some grated courgette or those fried shallots (readily available from Asian supermarkets) to sprinkle over the top of the cooked fritters or to include in the mixture.

Karen: Kumara is a colourful, nutritious vegetable that's full of antioxidants. It's a great source of fibre, contains Vitamins C and E, and beta-carotene, which is a form of Vitamin A.

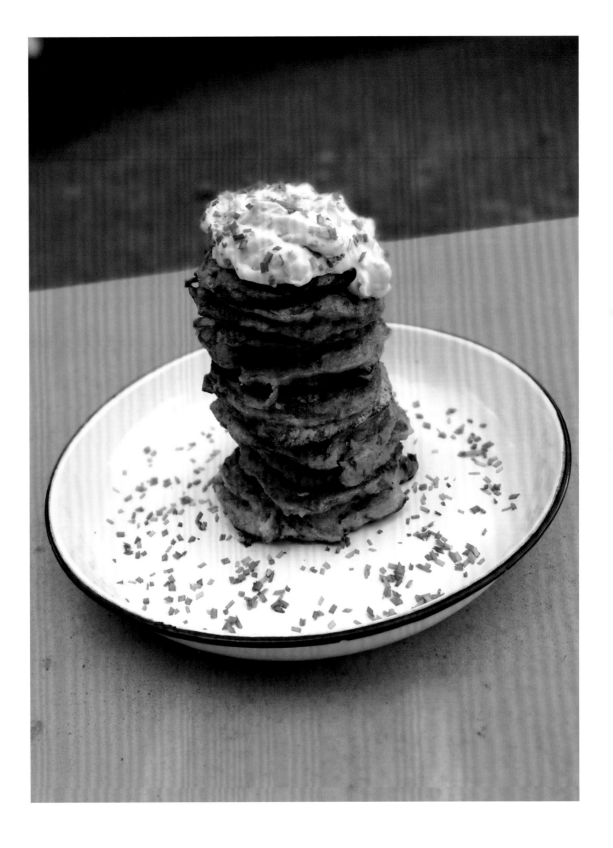

Mushrooms with Polenta and Salsa Verde

4–6   PREP: 10 min   COOKING TIME: 15 min   GF

SALSA VERDE:

4 tbsp finely chopped **parsley**

½ **shallot**, finely sliced

zest and **juice** of 1 **lemon**

1 tbsp good quality **white wine vinegar**

2 tbsp **olive oil**

salt and **pepper** to taste

MUSHROOMS:

50g (1.7oz) **butter**, plus a little extra

2 **shallots**, finely sliced

4 cloves **garlic**, finely sliced

several sprigs of **rosemary** and **thyme leaves** removed from stems

800g (28oz) mix of **mushrooms**, sliced (see note below)

½ cup (125ml) **dry white wine**

POLENTA:

5 cups (1250ml) good quality **chicken** or **vegetable stock**

1 cup (250ml) instant **polenta**

60g (2.1oz) **butter**

50g (1.7oz) **parmesan**

Make the Salsa Verde first. In a bowl combine all ingredients and whisk together with a fork. Set aside until required.

To make the mushrooms add the butter to a large, heavy-based pan over a medium-low heat and let it bubble up. Add the shallot, garlic and herbs and gently fry until the vegetables are soft and translucent and everything is smelling wonderful. Add a little more butter if you feel the need, then add the mushrooms. Cook them down gently for about 10 minutes, then pour in the white wine. Cook until it bubbles, then simmer for 5 minutes or so until it reduces by at least half. Season to taste and set aside to keep warm while you prepare the polenta.

To make the polenta, bring the stock to a simmer in a saucepan, then pour in the polenta, whisking as you pour. Continue to cook, stirring vigorously for 1–2 minutes so that it thickens. Add the butter and parmesan, remove from the heat, and keep stirring for another minute or so. Add a little more stock or hot water if you think it is too thick. Alternatively, if it is too runny, let it cook down for a little longer. It should be thick but still of pouring consistency. Season well with salt and pepper to taste.

To serve, I like to pour the polenta onto a large warmed platter, then spoon the mushrooms and salsa verde over the top, and let everyone share. Alternatively, you can plate individually.

Sam: I deliberately leave it open as to what type of mushrooms you use for this. Portobello, Swiss brown, enoki, oyster and even pine mushrooms are all reasonably available.

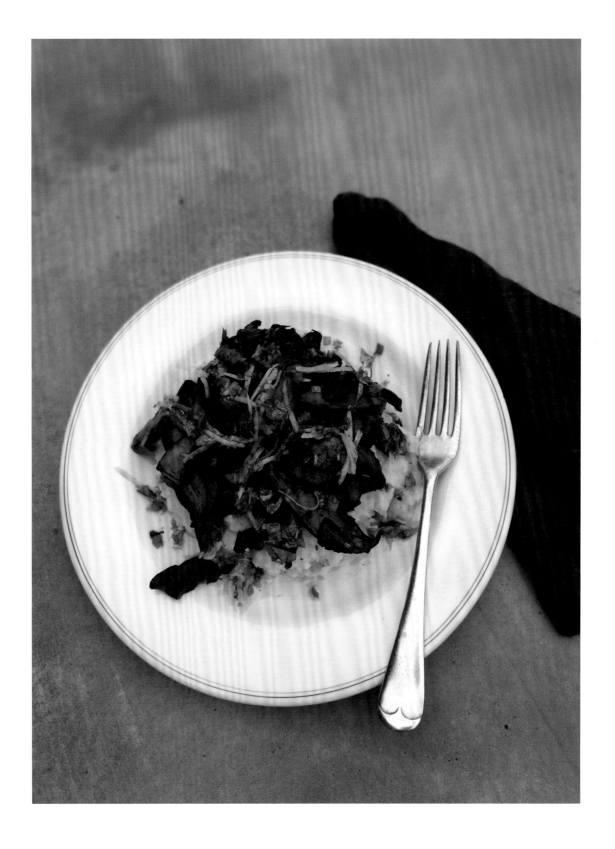

Spring Risotto of Asparagus, Broad Beans, Lemon & Feta

4–6   PREP: 15 min   COOKING TIME: 40 min    GF

INGREDIENTS:

200g (7oz) **broad beans**, either frozen or fresh

1 bunch fresh **asparagus**

1.5 litres good quality **chicken** or **vegetable stock**

50g (1.7oz) **butter**

1 **onion**, finely chopped

2 cloves **garlic**, finely chopped

250g (8.8oz) **aborio rice**

100ml **dry white wine**

zest and **juice** of 1 **lemon**

100g (3.5oz) **feta**

parmesan, to serve alongside

Pod the broad beans. If they are frozen, the best way to do this is to rinse them quickly under lukewarm water so that they are half defrosted but still firm inside, which means you can squeeze the broad bean out without squishing it into mush.

Remove and discard the woody stems from the asparagus and cut into 3cm lengths. Blanch in boiling water for 2 minutes, drain, and set aside.

Heat the stock nice and hot on top of the stove in an adjacent saucepan. In a large saucepan over a medium-low heat melt the butter. Add the onion and garlic, and cook gently for 6–7 minutes until soft and translucent. Add a little more butter if necessary. Stir the rice into the onion mixture so that the grains are coated in the butter. Increase the heat and add the white wine. Let it bubble and become absorbed into the rice before you add the first ladleful of stock to the mixture, stirring all the while. Continue to stir so that the bottom does not catch, and add the stock by the ladleful as it is absorbed until the rice is tender with the slightest bit of firmness in the middle, about 15–20 minutes. Taste and adjust the seasoning. Stir in the broad beans and asparagus, lemon zest and juice and combine well. Remove from the heat, crumble in the feta and stir it in.

Serve immediately with some parmesan on the side for people to grate in as they please.

Sam: Broad beans are a lovely thing. I know that the fresh ones, even when in season, are not always broadly (see what I did there) available, so the frozen ones are fine. Just remember that they need to be shelled. Use peas instead, if you like.

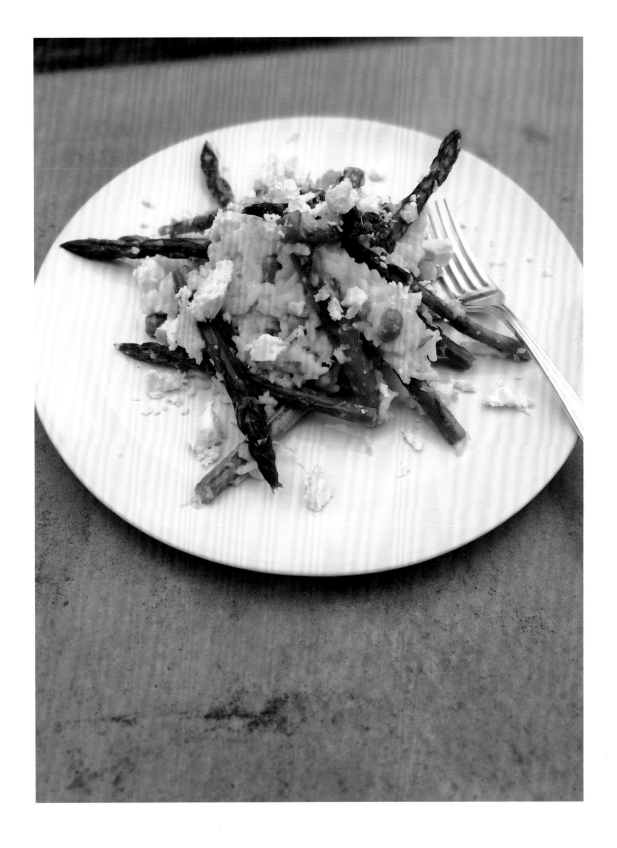

Moroccan Chicken with Preserved Lemon, Kumara and Spiced Yoghurt

4–6   PREP: 10 min   COOKING TIME: 40 min   GF

INGREDIENTS:

6 **chicken thighs**

½ **preserved lemon**, finely chopped

1 tsp **ground cinnamon**

1 tsp **cumin seeds**

olive oil

salt and **pepper**

1 tsp **ras el hanout**

1 **onion**, sliced

2 medium-size **kumara**, scrubbed and cut into 3cm chunks

2 **carrots**, cut into chunks

500ml **chicken stock**

1 x 400g (14oz) can **chickpeas**, well rinsed

½ cup (125ml) **unsweetened natural yoghurt**

1 tsp **ras el hanout**

a little chopped **mint** and **coriander** (use either or both)

Preheat the oven to 180°C. In a bowl combine the chicken thighs, preserved lemon, cinnamon and cumin seeds with about 1 tablespoon of olive oil and some salt and pepper to taste, and the ras el hanout. Set aside for a minute.

Get a wide, ovenproof pan over a medium heat. Add some olive oil and when it is hot add the onion. Cook for several minutes until the onion is soft. Add the kumara and carrot and cook for a few minutes until the vegetables are a little bit caramelised (you might need to add a little more olive oil if necessary), followed by the chicken thighs and all that comes with it. Cook the chicken for a minute or two on each sides so that it browns a little. Pour in the stock over the top of everything, add the drained chickpeas, and then pop the pan into the oven. Cook for 25–30 minutes or until the chicken is cooked through and tender, the kumara has softened, and the stock has reduced down a bit. Remove from the oven and set aside while you combine the yoghurt and ras el hanout with a little salt and pepper. Sprinkle the chopped coriander and mint over the top of the chicken and serve alongside the spiced yoghurt.

Sam: Traditionalists insist that twelve spices make a real ras el hanout, however, it varies enormously from region to region, with a good amount of fierce rivalry. I'm also a sucker for preserved lemon, another key Moroccan flavour. It is damn simple to make yourself. A little goes a long way, and it keeps a long time in the fridge – give it a go.

Karen: As well as being an easy and nutritious one-pan dish, the beauty of this recipe is that the spicy yoghurt can be served on the side, accommodating different tastes within a family.

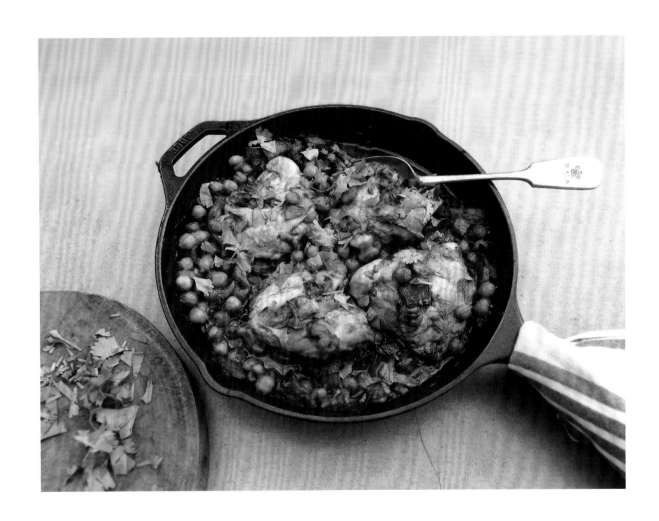

Polpette

4–6   PREP: 30 min   COOKING TIME: 75 min

INGREDIENTS:

olive oil

1 **onion**, peeled and finely chopped

2 cloves **garlic**, finely chopped

several sprigs of **rosemary**

2 tbsp **pine nuts**

salt and **pepper**

½ cup (25g/0.88oz) **fresh breadcrumbs**

500g (17.6oz) **pork mince**

200g (7oz) **ricotta**

1 **egg**

50g (1.7oz) grated **parmesan**

zest and **juice** of 1 **lemon**

small handful of **flat leaf parsley**, finely chopped

small handful of **oregano**

3 **tomatoes**

Get a frying pan over a moderate heat. Add about 2 tablespoons of oil, then stir in the onion and garlic. Cook gently for several minutes until soft and translucent, then strip the rosemary leaves off their woody stems and add to the mix along with the pine nuts. Continue to cook for a couple of minutes until the pine nuts turn golden brown. Season well and remove from the heat.

In a large mixing bowl combine the breadcrumbs, pork mince, ricotta, egg, two-thirds of the parmesan, lemon zest, parsley and the cooked onion mixture. Strip the leaves from half of the oregano, chop roughly, and mix in using your hands to combine everything thoroughly. Season bravely (pork mince requires a generous amount of salt), and then fry a little of the mixture off to check if it needs more salt or pepper. Adjust according to taste, then cover the bowl with cling film and place in the fridge for at least 1 hour (but overnight is even better).

About an hour before you want to serve them, remove the mix from the fridge. Using your hands (this is best done with wet hands), roll into smallish balls slightly larger than a walnut.

In a large frying pan over a moderate heat, add 2–3 tablespoons of olive oil and gently fry the meatballs, in batches if necessary, until they are nicely golden brown on all sides.

Finely chop the tomatoes. Preheat the oven to 200°C on fan grill. Arrange the meatballs on a roasting tray and scatter the chopped tomato over the top, followed by the remaining grated parmesan and oregano sprigs. Drizzle some olive oil over the top and grill in the oven for 6–10 minutes. Take care not to let them burn. After removing them from the oven, allow them to rest for 5 minutes before serving.

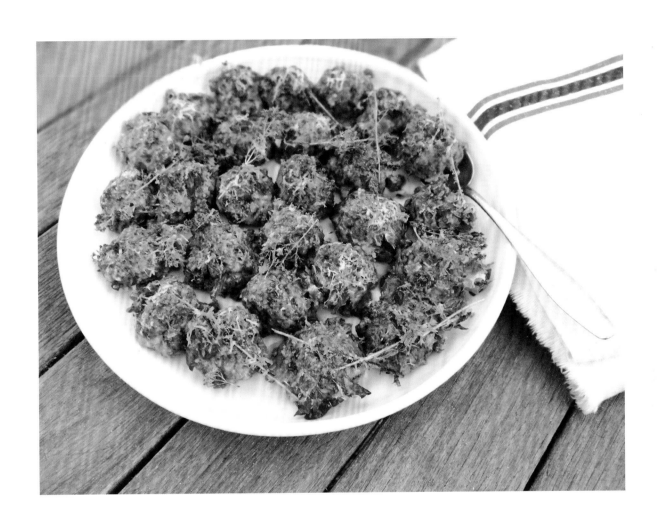

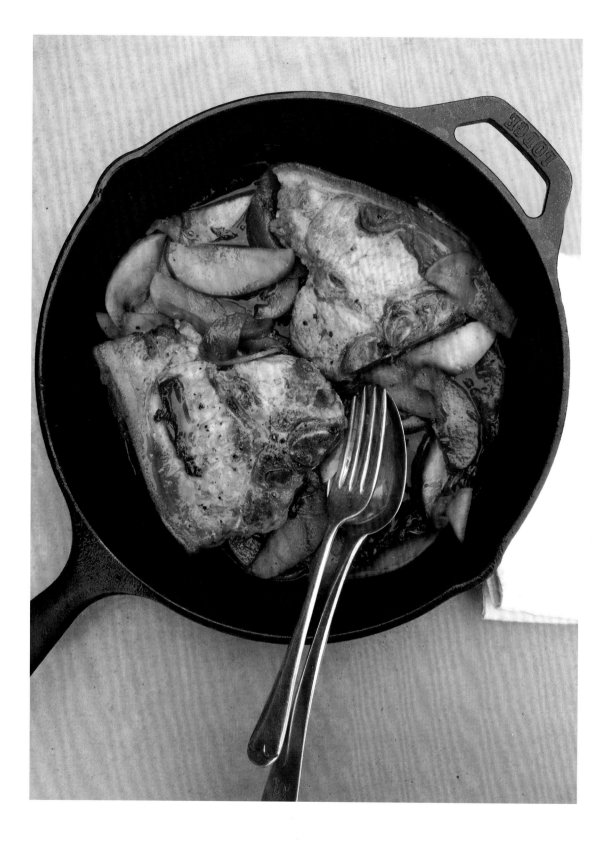

Pork Chops with Apple, Sage & Sweet Wine

◯ 2   PREP: 5 min   COOKING TIME: 10 min   GF

INGREDIENTS:

2 **pork loin chops** on the bone

salt and **pepper**

olive oil

1 tsp **butter**

1 **Braeburn apple**, cored and thinly sliced

small handful of **sage**, leave whole

1 tsp **wholegrain mustard**

1 cup (250ml) **sherry** or **sweet white wine**, eg riesling or pinot gris

Season the chops with salt and pepper on all sides.

Get a heavy pan going over a moderate heat and let it heat up for a minute or two. Add a bit of oil and butter and let it melt and sizzle up. Add the chops in the pan and cook for several minutes on each side and then the other, until they are nicely golden brown and no longer pink in the middle. Remove from the pan and transfer to a warm plate to rest. Add the apples to the same pan and cook them down for 1–2 minutes or so, adding a little more oil if the pan is too dry. Once the apples have softened a bit, stir in the sage and mustard, followed by the sherry or wine. Bring the heat up and let it bubble up and reduce down by half. Return the chops to the pan and nestle them into the sauce to coat. Season to taste, then serve.

Sam: The humble chop is perhaps a bit overlooked these days, but served with some fluffy, buttery mash alongside to catch all of those delicious juices it becomes a very tempting meal.

Karen: Pork has a number of important nutrients such as Vitamin B6 and B12, iron, magnesium, potassium and zinc. It's also a great source of protein.

Roast Pork Leg Stuffed with Courgette and Garlic

 6   PREP: 10 min   COOKING TIME: 150 min   GF   DF

INGREDIENTS:

3 **courgettes**, grated

4 cloves **garlic**, finely sliced

1 **red chilli**, deseeded and finely chopped (optional)

1 tbsp **Dijon mustard**

zest and **juice** of 1 **lemon**

salt and **pepper**

olive oil

1.5kg (532oz) **boned butterflied pork leg** or **shoulder**, skin on

Preheat the oven to 220°C on fan bake. Combine the grated courgette, sliced garlic, finely chopped chilli and mustard in a bowl. Add the zest and juice from the lemon, and salt and pepper to taste.

Spread the meat out, skin side down, and season well. Spread the stuffing over the top. Carefully roll the meat up firmly, but not so tightly that the stuffing starts to squeeze out everywhere. If this happens, just unroll it and try again. Secure each end with a couple of bamboo skewers so that it keeps together and place in a roasting dish. Score the skin with a sharp knife, rub a bit of olive oil into the skin and then sprinkle over a generous amount of sea salt and a few grinds of pepper. Pop in the oven and let it cook for 20 minutes at 220°C on fan bake, so that the skin starts to crisp up, then reduce the temperature to 170°C and cook for another 2 hours. If the crackling hasn't bubbled up and gone all crisp, give it 5 minutes or so under fan grill on high, but be sure to watch it like a hawk so that it doesn't burn.

Remove the pork from the oven and allow it to rest at for least 10 minutes under tin foil before serving. Soft polenta and some simply dressed leaves are all you need to sit alongside.

Sam: Not only does the flavour of courgette sit well alongside pork, it will also help to keep the meat from going dry. Add some torn up day-old bread to the stuffing to make it more substantial, or perhaps some bacon or caramelised onion.

Karen: This recipe is a fabulous flavourful dish for the family, but it can be served without the stuffing if less flavour is preferred.

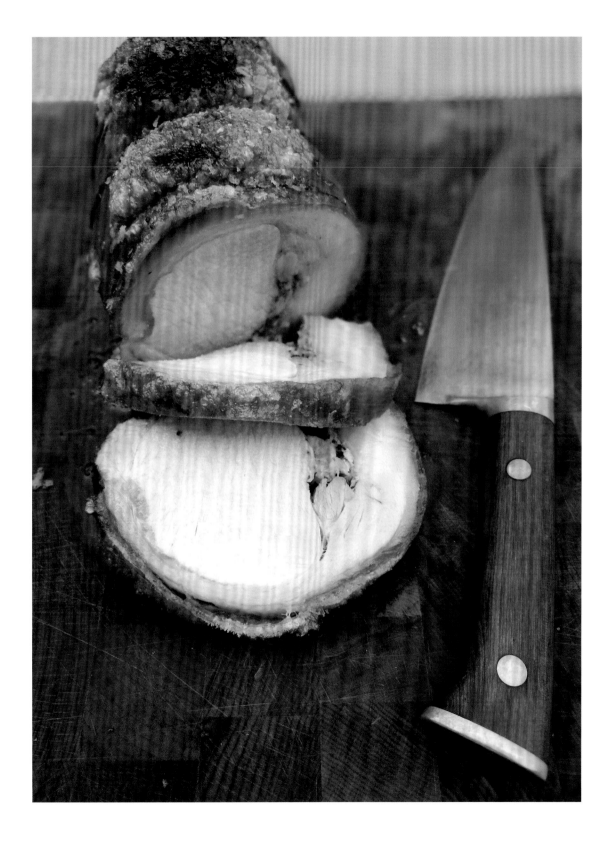

Curry of Pumpkin, Snake Beans, Cashews and Curry Leaves

4–6   PREP: 15 min   COOKING TIME: 60 min   DF

INGREDIENTS:

½ **crown pumpkin**, peeled, deseeded and cut into smallish pieces

vegetable oil

salt and **pepper**

1 **red onion**, peeled and sliced

2 tsp **cumin seeds**

1 tsp **ground coriander**

1 tsp **turmeric**

1 tsp **garam masala**

handful of **fresh curry leaves**

1 x 400ml can **coconut milk**

1 cup (150g/5.3oz) **roast cashew nuts**, plus a little extra

1 tbsp **soy sauce**

handful of **snake or green beans**, washed and cut into 8–10cm lengths

1 **lime**, quartered, to serve

1 **red chilli**, deseeded and finely chopped, to serve (optional)

brown rice, to serve

Preheat the oven to 180°C on fan bake.

Spread the pumpkin over an oiled roasting tray. Drizzle a little more oil over it and season well with salt and pepper. Roast in the oven for about 25–30 minutes until the pumpkin is tender and a little caramelised. Remove and allow to cool down.

In the meantime, place a large deep frying pan or saucepan over a moderate heat and add about 3 tablespoons of oil. When it has heated, add the onion and fry for several minutes until it has softened and become translucent. Add the cumin seeds, ground coriander, turmeric, garam masala and curry leaves and continue to fry for another minute until the spices are nice and fragrant (take care not to let them burn). Stir in the coconut milk, cashews and the soy sauce, and then let everything simmer for 5 minutes until the mixture has thickened and reduced. Carefully fold the cooled pumpkin and the beans into the mixture, then cook for another 3–4 minutes until the snake beans are just cooked, but still have a bit of crunch. Taste and season accordingly with salt and pepper, and serve.

Sam: Serve on or alongside brown rice, with a bit of lime juice squeezed over the top, and some finely chopped fresh chilli or chilli paste, if you fancy a bit of kick.

Karen: Another tasty recipe from Sam that puts you in charge of how hot or mild you want the finished dish to be.

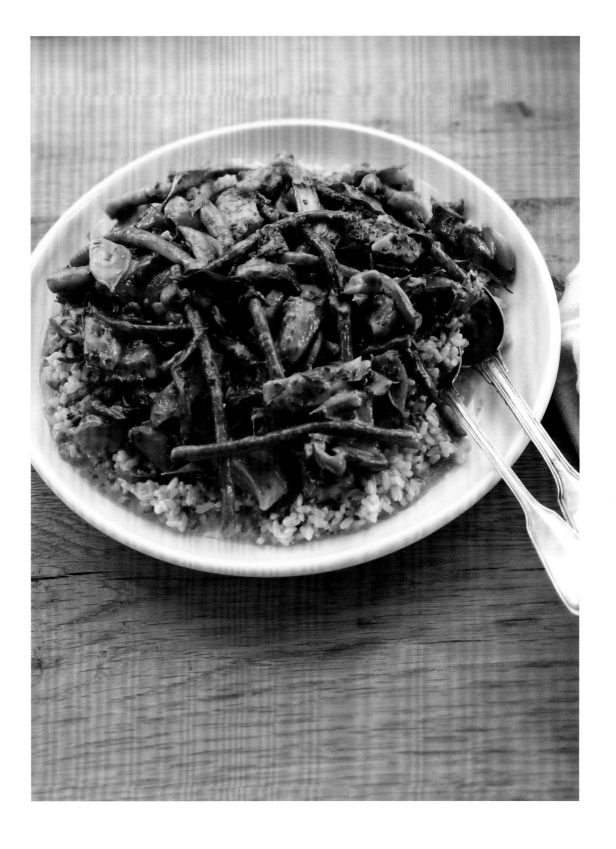

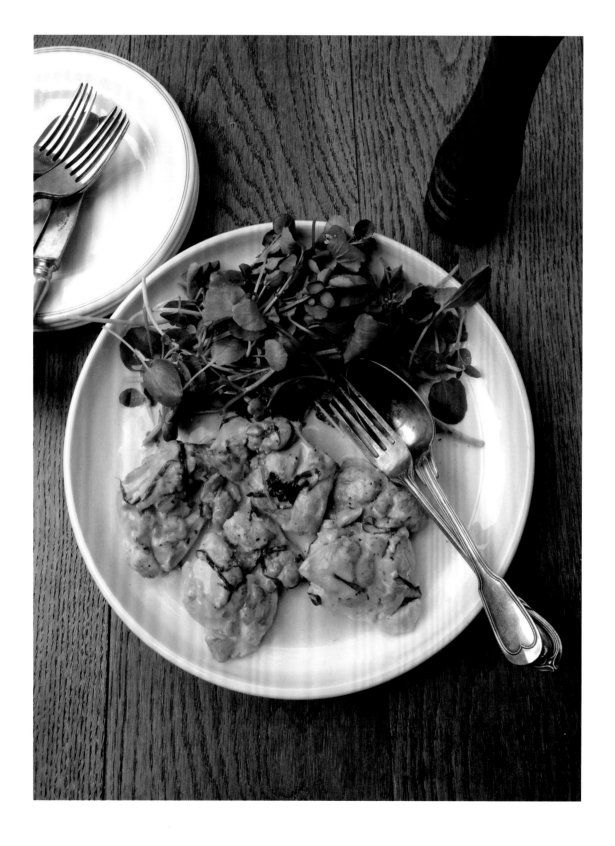

Tarragon Chicken

4–6   PREP: 5 min   COOKING TIME: 15 min

INGREDIENTS:

6 **chicken thighs**, boned and skinned

2 tbsp **plain flour**, for dusting

olive oil

salt and **pepper**

1 cup (250ml) **dry white wine**

small handful of **French tarragon leaves**, lightly chopped

½ cup (125ml) **cream**

Preheat the oven to 180°C.

Dust the chicken in the flour and season well. Get a large oven-proof pan going over a moderately high heat with a bit of oil. Shake any excess flour off the chicken, and add to the pan, in batches, if need be. Fry the pieces until golden brown on both sides, and then remove to a plate.

Add to the same pan the white wine and tarragon, and let the wine bubble up and reduce down a little. Stir in the cream, season well with salt and pepper, let everything bubble back up a bit, then return the chicken to the pan. Coat the pieces in the sauce, then pop the whole thing in the oven for 5 minutes or so until the chicken is cooked through and the sauce has reduced down a little. Taste and season if necessary, then serve.

Sam: This is one of my all time favourite comfort dishes. Make sure you buy French tarragon, as Russian tarragon is almost completely tasteless. Supermarkets should only ever sell the French stuff, but be a bit careful when you're at the garden centre as both varieties look the same, so make sure to check that it has that distinctive fragrance.

I don't really like to serve much else with this. Keep it simple. A couple of dressed leaves, and perhaps some steamed and buttered rice to soak up some of that glorious sauce.

Karen: Of Sam's wonderful recipes, this is definitely one of my all-time favourites. It's the subtle flavour of tarragon that makes it so special. Tarragon has loads of antioxidants, is great for digestion and it can help stimulate appetite in people who are feeling poorly.

Asparagus Frittata with Feta, Pine Nuts and Mint

 6   PREP: 5 min   COOKING TIME: 20 min   GF

INGREDIENTS:

2 tbsp **pine nuts**

olive oil

2 bunches **asparagus**, stems trimmed and cut into 3cm-long pieces

8 **eggs**

150g (5.3oz) **feta**

handful of **mint**, chopped

salt and **pepper**

zest of 1 **lemon**

Preheat the oven to 200°C on fan bake.

Get a heavy oven-friendly pan going over a low heat and gently toast the pine nuts until golden brown. Transfer to a plate and set aside. To the same pan add a tablespoon of olive oil and add the asparagus. Fry gently for 2–3 minutes just to cook them slightly, then remove to a plate as well. Keep the pan going over a medium-high heat.

Whisk up the eggs together well, then crumble in about half the feta, half the mint, some salt and pepper and the lemon zest. Mix everything through to combine. Add a little more olive oil to the pan and allow it to heat up. Pour in the egg mixture, then spread the asparagus evenly over the top, followed by the pine nuts. Cook for about 2 minutes, then place in the oven for about 10–15 minutes until the frittata is golden brown and cooked through.

Remove from the oven and allow to cool slightly for 5 minutes. Crumble the remaining feta and mint over the top. Slice into generous wedges and serve.

Sam: Frittata is an excellent way of using up leftovers; roasted vegetables, bacon, cheese and so on.

Karen: Asparagus is a low calorie food that is packed with vitamins and minerals, in particular Vitamin K that helps with bone density.

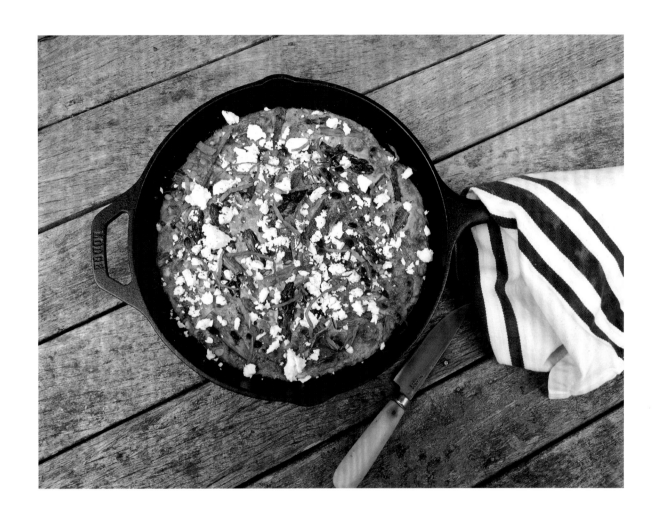

Omelette Arnold Bennett

 2   PREP: 5 min   COOKING TIME: 25 min

INGREDIENTS:

150ml **cream**

200ml **milk**

salt and **pepper**

1 **bay leaf**

200g (7oz) **smoked white fish**, eg haddock, kingfish or gemfish, flaked

2 tbsp **butter**

1 tbsp **flour**

5 **eggs**

parmesan

chopped **flat-leaf parsley** or **chives**, to serve

In a saucepan over a moderate heat combine the cream, milk, a little salt and pepper, bay leaf and the flaked smoked fish, and poach gently for about 10 minutes. Strain the fish from the liquid, reserving the liquid. In a separate saucepan melt half the butter over a low heat, then add the flour and cook over a low heat for 2 minutes. Gradually whisk in the reserved poaching liquid and allow the mixture to cook and thicken for another 5 minutes or so. Take off the heat. Beat one of the eggs and whisk into the mixture, then return the fish to the pan.

Preheat the oven grill to the highest setting. Beat together the remaining 4 eggs with a little salt and pepper.

Get a good oven-proof frying pan going over a high heat, then add the remaining butter and let it melt and sizzle. At this point, you can either make one large omelette or two smaller ones, in which case you would do the following in two batches: pour in the beaten egg and shake the pan around a bit, moving the runny egg around so that it spreads and cook. When the egg is almost cooked but still wobbly, pour the fish mixture over the egg, grate some parmesan over the top, then pop it under the grill and let it cook for several minutes until it is puffy and golden. Serve immediately, with some chopped parsley or chives and a little extra parmesan grated over the top.

Karen: A really simple, tasty meal this one, eggs are a great source of inexpensive, high quality protein, along with Vitamin B2, B6, B12, Vitamin D and the minerals zinc, iron and copper.

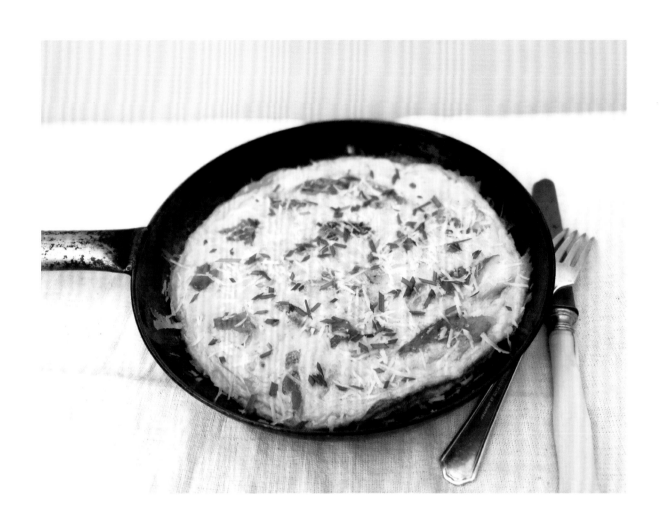

Rag Pasta with Pumpkin, Hazelnuts and Soft Cheese, and Sage Butter

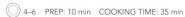 4–6   PREP: 10 min   COOKING TIME: 35 min

INGREDIENTS:

½ large **butternut pumpkin**, peeled and deseeded

olive oil

salt and **pepper**

200g (7oz) **lasagne sheets**

200g (7oz) **butter**

handful of **sage leaves**

100g (3.5oz) **soft white cheese**, eg ricotta, buffalo mozzarella or chévre

½ cup (75g/2.6oz) **toasted hazelnuts**, roughly chopped

Preheat the oven to 180°C.

Bring a large saucepan of salted water up to the boil. In the meantime, cut the pumpkin into crescents and add to an oiled baking dish. Season well with salt and pepper and roast in the oven for about 25 minutes until tender and a wee bit caramelised.

While the pumpkin is cooking, break the lasagne sheets into largish shards and drop into the simmering water. Cook until al dente, then drain well.

Melt the butter in a saucepan over a low heat until the white milk solids have separated out. Strain off the milk solids and discard, then return the clarified butter to the pan. Once it is quite hot, add the sage leaves and fry quickly until they are crisp.

On a warm platter arrange the cooked pasta and pumpkin and season everything well. Scatter the cheese and hazelnuts over, then lastly spoon the sage butter over and serve immediately.

Sam: The pumpkin, hazelnut and soft cheese combo is a crowd-pleasing winner, but you can fill the pasta with anything you like; sautéed mushrooms, spinach and ricotta or courgette, feta and lemon are all good alternatives.

Karen: The humble pumpkin is packed with fibre, and the beta-carotene is converted to Vitamin A in the body, making it a powerful antioxidant.

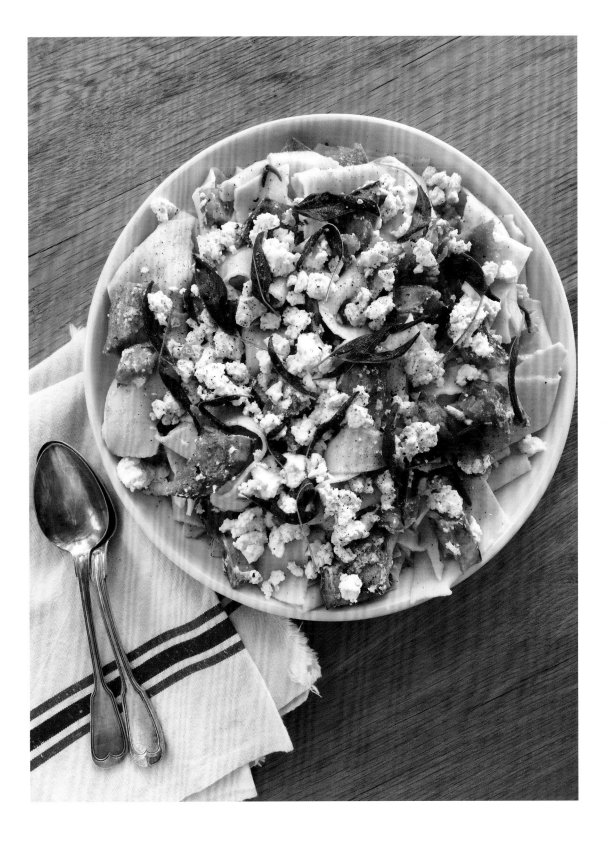

Wild Rice, Salmon, Edamame and Pickled Ginger

4–6   PREP: 10 min   COOKING TIME: 20 min    DF

INGREDIENTS:

400g (14.1oz) **wild rice**

500g (17.6oz) **fresh salmon,** pin-boned

olive oil

sea salt and **black pepper**

zest and **juice** of 1 **lime**

1 tbsp **sesame oil**

2 tbsp **soy sauce**

½ tsp **wasabi paste**

1½ cups (180g/6.3oz) **shelled edamame**

3 tbsp **pickled ginger**, roughly chopped

½ cup (101g/3.5oz) **mung beans**

handful of **bean sprouts** or **microgreens**

small handful of **coriander leaves**

Preheat the oven to 200°C.

Wash the rice several times under cold water, drain, and place in a saucepan with two and a half times as much water. Leave to simmer, covered, for about 15 minutes over a medium heat, topping up with more water if necessary until the rice is just tender. Rinse under cold water and drain well.

In the meantime, drizzle the salmon with a little olive oil, season with salt and pepper and roast in the oven for about 20 minutes until it is cooked to your liking. Allow to cool a little.

In a wee bowl combine the lime zest and juice, sesame oil, soy sauce and wasabi paste and mix well into a dressing.

Combine the cooked rice with the edamame, chopped ginger, mung beans and the dressing mixture. Taste and season accordingly. Break the cooked salmon into chunks and fold carefully into the mixture. Scatter the bean sprouts and coriander over the top and serve.

Karen: Mung beans are a very filling food, high in protein, fibre and minerals and Vitamin B. In this recipe you get great taste and nutrition.

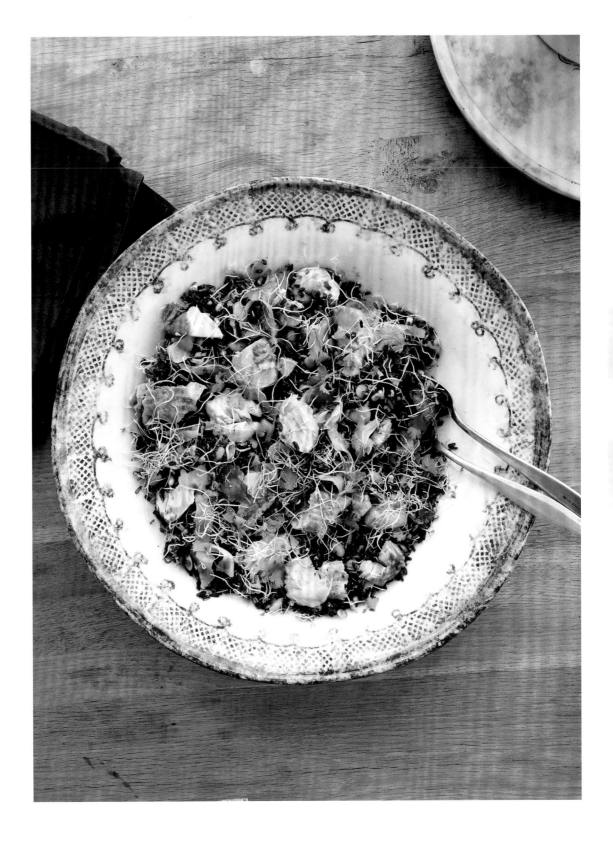

Hair Care

ADVICE FROM EXPERTS AROUND HAIR LOSS & HAIR REGROWTH

'Hair loss was an expected side effect of my treatment so before it started I shaved it all off. Being bald has been liberating and eye-opening. I am currently in the regrowth phase.' – Amber

'Hair loss must be especially hard for young women whose long tresses are so much part of their sex appeal and femininity. It's a challenge, even for older women like me.' – Lindsey

Losing your hair when undergoing chemotherapy is undoubtedly a challenging experience. But it doesn't need to be as devastating as it might initially seem. By implementing some practical strategies there are ways to get through this difficult time with your head held high and still feeling good about yourself, confident in the knowledge that eventually your hair will grow back.

Suzanne Wolton, who owns Jessica's Wig and Beauty Salon regularly helps people with choosing wigs after losing their hair to chemotherapy, as well as alopecia, illness or age. Her business provides an invaluable service for people who, whatever their circumstances, are facing hair loss in their community.

CHOOSING THE PERFECT WIG

The first piece of advice from Suzanne is to organise a wig for yourself earlier rather than later on. Don't wait until you have lost your hair. By being prepared, you can minimise the trauma.

'Ideally anyone that wants to get a wig close to their own hair colour and style should come to see us before starting chemotherapy so we can see what their hair looks like. If they come in later then we can't tell. And while that doesn't stop us from finding something that suits them, some people want the comfort of knowing they can have exactly what they used to have. Even if they want to go for a different look, it's better to organise a wig before treatment when they are feeling better.'

So are there any rules for choosing a wig? Suzanne is adamant that there are no rules except getting the correct size and choosing one they feel really good about wearing.

'Some people want a wig as close as possible to their existing hair. Whereas others use this challenging time as an opportunity to try something new. We helped a lady a couple of weeks ago who went for a very vibrant red colour and she looked amazing. She just felt that she wanted to go with something that makes a statement.'

I ask if people are better going for lighter colours when they are unwell.

'Intuitively, you would say yes,' said Suzanne. 'But in practice what I see is that a lot of people suit darker-coloured wigs. Overall, it's about half and half. Matching your eyebrow colour is a good way to achieve a natural look, but there are no rules. You could try to make it very scientific, but at the end of the day, it's a relaxed personal choice.

'We don't push people into making a choice. Even if we think that a particular wig looks great, but the customer prefers something else, that's just fine. However, we wouldn't let people walk out the door looking odd; there is a fine line between the customer always being right and our expertise, so we just try to steer them a little bit.

'At the moment, long straight styles are very popular, along with short pixie cuts. Wig manufacturers change their range of styles every two to three years so that people can keep up with the trends if they choose.

'The most important thing about a wig is the confidence it can give an individual. Choosing one can also be a fun experience and we encourage people to bring their friends and have some fun with them. We've had groups where everyone tries on wigs, and it is a great opportunity to take photos to send to loved ones who can't be with them. Just for fun, we have a Tammy Wynette style of wig, which people like trying on for fun – we see it as a silver lining at a time like this.'

LOOKING AFTER YOUR WIG

'Looking after a synthetic wig is pretty simple. They are easier to take care of in my view, and not as expensive as human hair wigs. They also hold their style, making them perfect for people who want something that is always ready to wear. Alongside our wigs, you can buy a special wig shampoo. Alternatively, put a capful of very mild shampoo in some cold water and gently wash it, then rinse it equally gently. Don't wring it or squeeze it, let it dry naturally. As for how often you wash it, this depends on how exerted you feel, but on average don't wash it more than once every three weeks.'

PREPARING FOR YOUR HAIR TO FALL OUT

I spoke with trichologist and hair stylist Nigel Russell to see what advice he could offer. With 30 years' experience in the hairdressing industry and as a certified trichologist (ie, he's qualified in the scientific study of the health of hair and scalp) for the last 18 years, he knows more than most about the subject. Nigel also created the Holistic Hair products range and he consults to the Seville's salon group.

As we talked, Nigel stressed the importance of people having a good relationship with their hairdresser during this time.

'You need someone who has empathy with what you are going through. To begin with, I usually suggest cutting long hair, but gradually, not all at once, to minimise the trauma of losing it. Some women will hang on to their long hair for as long as they possibly can out of fear, but it really is best to gradually get it shortened, probably between the shoulder and the neck, before you start to lose it.

'Think about asking your hairdresser to give you a chic medium to short haircut that emphasises your cheekbones and which gives you soft lines through the cheeks and the chin. Ideally your hair should still cover your forehead as that is where it is going to be looking the thinnest, so either a fringe or side fringe is a good idea. And if you decide to change the shape or colour, choose a shape and colour to suit not just your skin tone, but also to make you feel good. However, a very short cropped, gamine or pixie cut will always be the least traumatic when you start losing your hair. So do it in gradual stages is my advice. Even if you are attached to your long hair, you can gradually wean yourself off your long hair. But with the view of growing it longer when you are well, of course.'

HAIR CARE AFTER CHEMOTHERAPY

Through his vast experience, Nigel has invaluable advice regarding future hair care after finishing chemotherapy, but as he explained it helps to understand how chemotherapy changes the hair follicle.

'The actual follicle changes shape from round to oval after chemotherapy, which causes the hair to curl. I've seen it for myself under a microscope. So that is why 90 per cent of people's hair turns curly after chemo, however over time it returns to its normal state.

'When it grows back it will be lanugo hair, which is like the fine hair that is sometimes found on the body of a newborn baby. It needs to be treated gently so ideally use chemical-free shampoo at this time which will also help protect your scalp, which is likely to be very sensitive.

'It takes time for the hair to recover after chemotherapy. As the toxins leave the body, there is also a loss of pigment. So although the colour of your hair will initially change, it will gradually return to its previous colour. But the lack of pigment will cause it to absorb all the light, and it will feel more frizzy and dry.'

'After chemotherapy, it may take some time for the hair to regrow and remembering that the shape of the follicle becomes altered to an oval pattern, so the new hair predominantly will be fine and frizzy then becoming curly and eventually back to normal. To aid the regrowth, it is imperative to use natural non-sensitising, chemical-free products. And although there are many products on the market that profess to encourage hair growth, watch out for those that are chemically formulated as they should be avoided in the early stages of recovery.'

Nigel recommends gentle head massages on a regular basis as they will aid the recovery process and are also a form of pampering, which is good for the soul.

'Never use essential oils undiluted on your hair or scalp; they should be blended into a carrier oil. The best carrier oils for encouraging hair growth are sweet almond, coconut, macadamia, jojoba, castor and Vitamin E, while essential oils known to stimulate blood flow to the follicle include lavender, rosemary, cedarwood, palma rosa and chamomile.'

Here are a couple of soothing massage oil 'recipes' for the scalp. In both cases the ratio of essential oils to the carrier oil should be 5 drops to 10ml and they should always be mixed in a glass bottle as essential oils interact with plastic with unpleasant results. Shake well before application and always do a patch test before using either of these blends for the first time to ensure you are not sensitive to any of the fragrances. You can do this by massaging in a few drops behind one of your ears. Leave for half an hour, then check that your skin is not red or itchy.

Using a 200ml glass bottle with either a dropper-type lid or a flip top, mix up a blend of 100ml castor oil, 50ml coconut oil and 40ml macadamia oil. Add 20 drops of lavender, 15 drops of cedarwood and 5 drops of rosemary

oil. Let it sit for at least 1 hour or preferably overnight before using.

Again, using a 200ml glass bottle with either a dropper-type lid or a flip top, mix up a blend of 100ml sweet almond oil, 60ml jojoba oil and 30ml Vitamin E oil. Add 20 drops of lavender, 15 drops of palma rosa and 5 drops of chamomile oil. Let it sit for at least 1 hour or preferably overnight before using. Shake well before application. Note: this is a milder mix for when the hair has started to grow a bit.

Whichever combination you are using, use on a dry, unwashed scalp as water will slow down the absorption. Begin by applying several large drops into the palm of the hand, then dip the fingers of the other hand into the palm and use them to rub the oil into the scalp, starting from the crown. Remember more is not necessarily better, so use sparingly. You do not need to saturate or apply too much oil; just enough to avoid any friction on the skin. Wipe away any excess so none gets in your eyes.

Using both hands, massage in a circular motion to encourage blood flow and allow the oils to penetrate into the scalp. A massage can be anywhere from 10 to 20 minutes, depending on how much time/energy you have. Ideally, ask your partner or a friend to massage your scalp – it will be a nice experience for both of you.

Leave the oils on your scalp for anywhere between 1 hour and overnight; cover your head with a shower cap or towel to keep in the warmth.

When it is time to remove the oils, gently rub a small amount of a natural shampoo over your scalp (this is necessary because oil and water do not mix) before jumping in the shower to rinse it all out. If some hair has begun to grow then repeat with a second small amount of shampoo to ensure all the oil is washed out.

Note: This treatment can be repeated two or three times a week.

Follow-up

Nigel recommends using a water-based finishing rinse, with apple cider vinegar and essential oils, up to three times per week as it will tone the scalp and return the delicate pH balance to the correct, slightly acid state. It's best not to use commercial shampoos as most are more alkaline, which can lead to a dry or itchy scalp. A finishing rinse can be used three times per week.

He also has some invaluable advice for what to do – and what not to do – with your hair as it is growing out.

'Firstly, regarding colouring, you shouldn't do anything until your hair is at least 6cm long. I recommend a semi-permanent colour at this stage if you are concerned about chemicals as it doesn't change hair structure or colour permanently. This kind of colour treatment also has the bonus of giving a good reflection. If you want to use bleach, combine it with some essential oils, which will create volume.'

'Regarding cutting your hair, it's important to understand that the hair will be growing back at the same rate all around the head. It'll be shapeless, so make sure that your chosen hairstyle is cut close to the nape, ears, and the widest part of the head. You want to create height and volume, rather than just wispy edges. Consider creating a fringe or sweeping a fringe to the side as this will be the most flattering. Emphasise the cheekbones; it doesn't really matter what is happening at the back. If it is short at the back and longer at the front, you can grow your hair back from this style without too much angst.

'The regrowth curls last about six months before the hair starts to return to normal so keep a bit of shaping going on during this time. As a general rule, I suggest that people keep wearing their wig until their hair is about half the length of the wig, and then that could be the time to take it off.'

Nigel mentioned that as some of his clients who had long hair before their treatment now prefer their short locks, it pays to keep an open mind about what kind of hairstyle you might have when your hair returns to normal. Just like choosing a wig, there are no rules – just opt for something that suits you and gives you confidence.

'One of my clients is a classic example of this. She'd always had long hair, but after chemotherapy she decided on a very funky pixie white-blonde textured haircut. She had never had a short haircut but then, after chemo, she discovered it suited her. She now loves it, and everyone comments on it all the time. She says it was a bit of a blessing in disguise, as she would never have had it cut short if she hadn't had cancer.'

GENERAL HAIR CARE ADVICE

Not everyone loses their hair when going through cancer treatments, but hair can become thin, brittle and dry during this time. Nigel has advice for looking after your hair at this time.

'Focus on foods that are good for the liver. During cancer treatments, the liver takes a caning, so whatever happens to the liver happens to the hair. Choose good protein and iron-rich food in your diet such as eggs, fish, lean red meat and lots of vegetables.

'If you are passionate about getting your hair back to normal, minimise your intake of processed food and refined sugar. Whole food, real food, will always support healthy skin and hair. And remember to drink lots of water. In terms of supplements, always check with your oncologist, but you could consider a good slow-release multi Vitamin B, Vitamin C, omega-3 and silica.'

Nigel warns against any hair treatments that seem too good to be true as he says there is a lot of misguided information about the theories and the treatment that is needed to make hair regrow.

'I would caution against signing up for a long-term treatment that involves going to a specialist on a weekly basis, and which involves applying certain types of products to the scalp. There is no medical or scientific evidence that supports most of these treatments, so before signing up for such a thing seek advice from someone who is not only impartial but has some knowledge. People who have lost their hair tend to be very vulnerable and will often sign up

for a "silver bullet" treatment that offers their hair back sooner rather than later.

'Advances will be made in the future in stem cell therapy because science has already discovered there is a stem cell bulge along the hair bulb itself. Once they figure out how to stimulate it that will be the breakthrough for hair regrowth. But at the moment it is still being worked on, so my advice is to be very cautious about any advice you receive relating to miracle hair loss cures that sound too good to be true.'

Loss of eyelashes

It is common for people undergoing chemotherapy to lose their eyebrows and eyelashes. If you are concerned about this, ask your doctor about bimatoprost.

In a year-long trial, researchers at Southampton General Hospital and St Louis University in the USA analysed the effects of a daily application of bimatoprost to the upper eyelids of patients with poor eyelash growth as a result of recent chemotherapy. Bimatoprost was shown to be a safe and effective treatment for eyelash growth over a sustained period. For women especially losing their eyelashes can have an adverse effect on their psychological wellbeing, so bimatoprost is a viable option indeed.

In the meantime, however the clever use of eyeliner can be used to recreate the effect of eyelashes. Use an eyeliner pencil to apply a thin line along your upper and lower eyelids, then soften and slightly smudge the line with a cotton bud. False eyelashes are, of course, another option.

Loss of eyebrows

The absence of eyebrows can change the look of your face as they normally frame the face. If your brows become thin, use an eyebrow pencil in a suitable shade to fill in the gaps using short, light strokes.

In the event of having to create new brows altogether, study old photographs of yourself to find the position where your brows would normally arch. Using an eyebrow pencil, place a dot on that place, then draw another dot just above the brow bone, and a third one dot at the outside edge of where the eyebrow would normally finish. Use short strokes to connect the dots to create a brow line. With practice, you will find this no more difficult than putting on lipstick.

All of the recipes in this book will help with healthy hair, but of particular benefit are:

- Salmon, Buckwheat, Fennel, Capers and Dill, page 64
- Wild Rice, Salmon, Edamame and Pickled Ginger, page 122

Skin Care & Nails

STRATEGIES FOR KEEPING THEM IN GOOD CONDITION

'Chemotherapy has such a devastating effect on one's appearance. I remember driving home and pulling down the mirror and noticing I had more lines. It seemed like my face was cracking up.'
— Robyn

'I started hormone therapy, and within three weeks I could see a negative impact on my skin. It's very much the opposite of all those skin care adverts claiming you'll have better skin in 21 days!' — Joanna

Skin can certainly take a hammering during cancer treatment. Nutrition consultant and registered nurse Wendy Hamilton from Optimum Health and Nutrition has some good ideas about how to keep your skin in the best possible condition during this time. She recommends that you carefully read the labels of any cosmetics you might be using to check what's in them as some of them can be a toxic source of chemicals. It may be that you want to switch to using natural products.

'Rosehip is perfect for rehydrating dry skin, while silica is important for healthy hair as well as skin. And because silica is not always present in significant amounts in the soil in which our food is grown, you might want to take a supplement or investigate how to best use the herb horsetail, which contains silica. From your diet, look to food like leeks, green beans, chickpeas, celery, strawberries and asparagus.

'Zinc is important for skin and hair repair. It is best absorbed from animal sources, but it is also present in nuts such as Brazil nuts, and seeds like pumpkin seeds. Oysters are an excellent source of zinc, as well as scallops and other shellfish. However, when people aren't well, it might be useful to use supplements, as they are not digesting their food as well.'

Wendy advocates staying away from processed foods, and instead looking to real whole food to keep your skin looking as healthy as possible.

'Vitamin A is good for skin and can be found in food as diverse as liver, carrots, sweet potatoes, oranges, kale, melon, spinach, and apricots. A good quality purified cod liver oil could also be a good investment as it will provide Vitamin A

along with omega-3. Vitamin C is great for skin, and don't forget Vitamin D for your immune system, which we get mostly from being outdoors in sunshine, but it is also present in fatty foods like butter.'

Another person with valuable advice for skin care during and following cancer treatment is Megan Dempsey, a registered nurse with a Bachelor of Nursing degree. Previously a breast cancer nurse specialist, she is now an advanced clinical skin care specialist. We talk about overall skin care first. As well as a healthy diet, now there is good topical skin care available that can also improve your skin.

'There is currently a real move away from cosmetics that look lovely in their packaging and have a little bit of everything in them, but nothing active enough to make a difference. Discerning customers are moving to clinically proven active skin care from trained professionals. Skin is our single biggest organ, so we should all think about what we put on it. Personally, I see dry skin as a wounded skin.'

Megan tells me that active skin care has flipped the classic cleanse, tone and moisturise that people have thought was good skin care in the past. These days it is about using active skin care – usually in the form of serums that reach down into the basal layer to help the cells stay hydrated, plumped and dewy. And the good news is it is never too late.

Skin renews on average every 28 days, and Megan assures me that if you are on good topical vitamin skin care you should see a difference in two weeks – and it's all as simple as 'A, B, C'.

THE ABCS – AND MORE – OF GOOD SKIN CARE

Vitamin A, an oil-soluble vitamin, is the gold standard vitamin for all ageing skin concerns becase it:

- stimulates cell renewal and exfoliation

- smooths and refines fine lines and wrinkles, reduces hyperpigmentation and minimises pore size

- stimulates collagen and hyaluronic acid

- strengthens blood vessels

- is suitable for anyone concerned with ageing and it works for all skin types.

- Note: Vitamin A should be used in the evening.

Vitamin B3 niacinamide is a water-soluble vitamin that energises the cells, and brightens and boosts the health of the skin. It is ideal for:

- improving the health of all skin conditions, especially dry and impaired sensitive skin
- calming and strengthening, stimulating collagen and hyaluronic acid, and controlling oil flow
- hydrating and increasing the skin's natural moisturising factor
- repairing the skin's barrier function.

In summary, this vitamin brightens, balances and boosts the skin.

Vitamin C, another water-soluble vitamin, is essential for producing collagen and also:

- is an important antioxidant in controlling UV damage to cells
- inhibits inflammation within our cells, therefore assisting in the prevention of hyperpigmentation and ageing
- is recommended for the healing of scars.

Vitamin E, an oil-soluble vitamin, is one of the most potent antioxidants and is recommended for all skins to help protect the skin cell membranes from future damage. Further, it is:

- extremely protective, which is why it helps to protect wounds
- fabulous at protecting the barrier of the skin to assist in the hydrating process
- often used in combination with Vitamin C to get the most potent antioxidant protection.

Sunblock

There are two types of sunblock – chemical and physical. To protect your skin, Megan recommends you choose a physical sunblock with 30 SPF protection.

'Ignore products that claim to have 80–100 SPF as it just encourages people to leave it on the skin for longer, even though it doesn't offer any more protection. Good old-fashioned micronised zinc is the best and can very easily be added to tinted face lotions to avoid looking too white. Zinc is also very calming.

'I think of the sun as a big ball of radiation with UVA and UVB rays. Anywhere where there is natural light, even if you are indoors, you will be exposed to UVA radiation, so it's important to use a good SPF30 all-year round. On average people only need about 15–20 minutes of UV exposure a day to get enough Vitamin

D, which they will get from being out and about through hands, décolletage and things like that.'

Skin care nasties

Avoid skin care products that contain some or any of the following:

- Sodium lauryl sulphate

- Propylene glycol

- Formaldehyde

- Parabens or harsh preservative systems

- Hydroquinone

- Alcohol

- Mineral or petroleum-based oils

The packaging can tell you quite a lot. If the product claims to have active ingredients it should be protected from light, air and extreme temperatures, thus stay away from products in clear glass or plastic packaging. And avoid products which you have to dip your finger in to get access to it.

CHEMOTHERAPY

Take steps to have your skin in the best possible condition before you begin chemo treatment, which will affect every single cell in the body.

Megan recommends using topical Vitamin A, Vitamin C and Vitamin B, which does an excellent job of hydrating the skin.

'Vitamin B is amazing; it strengthens the cell walls to stop water loss in a very simplistic way because although you can drink water until the cows come home, if your cells are unable to hold the water it's not much help. Vitamin B also helps brighten the skin and evens the tone. It is one thing on the market that is good for skin types that are oily and dry, and everything in between. A dry skin can become an impaired skin and then it turns to cracked skin and then you have a wound. It's really important to keep your skin hydrated before starting chemotherapy. Choose a water-based cream without any nasties in it such as aqueous cream or lanolin, which is a naturally occurring cream that creates a good barrier, although some people are allergic to it, so it's not for everyone. Cleansers are very important, too, but avoid those that strip your skin of its natural oils. Stay away also from scrubs containing any kind of granules as they can cause microscopic cuts on the skin.'

When going through chemotherapy, stop using Vitamin A or any other active skin care, and look instead to skin care that has hydrates like hyaluronic, which is very calming and hydrating and which can be found in a lot of skin care ranges.

'Vitamin A is very anti-ageing, and it basically stimulates the nucleus of the cell to behave like a young cell, but it is best not to use it during chemotherapy treatment because it's important to avoid anything that may irritate the skin. Instead I suggest combining a pure hyaluronic cream (which has powerful anti-aging properties and is also one of the premier hydrating ingredients for skin) with Vitamin B in an appropriate form. But do ensure there is no perfume or other "nasties" present. As for Vitamin C products, some contain up to 8 per cent which for most people going through chemo will be too strong. Choose a product with about 4 per cent Vitamin C instead – a nice low dose keeps the cells hydrated and is especially good mixed with some hyaluronic and Vitamin E dual anti-oxidants. Stop using any active washers and replace with more creamy cleansers. In short, use products that aren't stripping away your natural oils.'

After chemotherapy your skin may be sensitised for one to two months, so Megan recommends visiting a skin care expert before reverting to your usual skin care routine.

RADIOTHERAPY

Keep your skin well hydrated and avoid all fragrances, much the same as you would if undergoing chemotherapy. Megan recommends using a pure aqueous cream, also a pH neutral aloe vera lotion. Avoid talcum powder, perfumes, and products containing alcohol or oil. And choose an aluminium-free stick or roll-on deodorant. These days when going through radiotherapy it is likely you will have a cling film dressing.

'This absorbs the effects of the radiation on the skin. It is like a plastic wrap and it will stay on during the radiation. In the old days radiation treatment used to be very traumatic on the skin, but it's now a lot less traumatising, and the impact of discolouration and pigmentation is much reduced. Look after your skin. As we know, it's our biggest organ and it needs lots of care. By keeping your skin hydrated during and after treatment you can avoid it cracking, which can lead to infection and delay recovery.'

After radiotherapy, water-based creams are better and kinder to your skin than oil-based products. And it is important to realise that the effects of radiation do not stop when the treatment has finished; the effect on your skin may well be worse for a month or so afterwards. This is because radiation has a cumulative effect.

'You put out fire with water, not oil. Similarly with a burn (ie radiation), oil can *increase the intensity, so water-based products are best, especially pH neutral aloe vera, which is also naturally cooling.'*

SURGERY

It can really make a difference if you are as fit and healthy as possible before surgery. As for taking supplements, do follow any recommendations made by your surgeon.

'Surgeons don't want you to take high doses of Vitamin C before surgery because it can make you bleed more than usual. Other supplements like fish oil and arnica should also be avoided for reasons your surgeon can explain so pay close attention to all his or her instructions.'

Megan has worked with many plastic surgeons, which is how she knows that the wound is usually taped for six to 12 weeks after surgery.

'Because scar tissue is only 70–80% as strong as skin, tape helps support healing by keeping the scar flat. The brown hypoallergenic tape used by surgeons can cope with getting a little bit wet, but dry it after your shower to avoid it getting soggy, which can lead to infection. Change the tape every two to three days, or sooner if it starts peeling off.'

There are different levels of scarring, so it is very individual for people.

'Some people with darker skin are prone to forming brown scars, and even just a bump can cause hyperpigmentation. Some fair skins might get raised pink scars. But keloid scars, which are caused by overgrowth of the scar tissue that develops around a wound, are a whole other issue. People usually know if they are prone to these because they form quite a lump, and are almost tumour-like. If you have a history of keloid scarring, discuss alternative dressings with your surgeon as it may be appropriate to use a slow-release silicone dressing to minimise the scarring.'

The key thing to remember is that scars can take up to two years to heal, so the look of your scar at a three or six-month mark is not representative of the future. Megan thoroughly endorses the use of Vitamin E to help the healing process.

'I am a great fan of massaging pure Vitamin E into the scar once taping the wound is no longer necessary because the skin has knitted together is and flat. Choose a pure Vitamin E and look for a product free of parabens and perfumes. Regular gentle massages will over time increase the blood flow and break up scar tissue.'

HORMONE TREATMENT

Hormonal therapy, like menopause, can have a dramatic effect on a woman's skin.

Again, Megan recommends reassessing your usual skin care regime so you can get the best possible anti-ageing results.

'You want to stop the clock by using a good sunblock, and then use active skin care to strengthen, hydrate and anti-age the skin as well as introducing topical Vitamin A, B and C into your skin care routine.'

NAILS

Chemotherapy will affect your nails to the extent that you may notice a line or ridge that effectively traces the cycle. However, these ridges are not permanent and will disappear in about six months. Other changes to your nails include brittleness and they may also become pigmented or discoloured. Follow these tips to keep your nails as healthy as possible:

- Keep your nails short; imperfections will not be as noticeable.

- Soak your fingers and toes in a bowl of undiluted white vinegar for five minutes; this is an easy and efficient way of improving your nails.

- Massage cuticle cream into the cuticle area daily to prevent dryness, splitting and hangnails.

- Avoid conventional nail polishes as they may contain toxic chemicals (water-based polish is a good alternative).

- Don't wear fake nails as they can trap bacteria which may cause infection.

- Alert your doctor to any signs of inflammation or infection.

All of the recipes in this book will help with healthy skin and nails, but of particular benefit are:

- Salmon, Buckwheat, Fennel, Capers and Dill, page 64

- Wild Rice, Salmon, Edamame and Pickled Ginger, page 122

Emotional Wellbeing

TIPS FOR THE DAYS YOU FEEL BLUE

'Surround yourself with good people and always have something to look forward to, eg lunch and dinner dates, trips, outings, catch-ups, movies – fun things you like.' — Jessica

'As well as support from wonderful family and friends, it was losing myself in my creative pursuits that helped me through this difficult time.' — Leigh

When you are dealing with cancer your emotional and spiritual wellbeing is as vital as your physical wellbeing. Positivity is important and will help how you experience things on a day-to-day basis, but it's important to keep things real and allow yourself to feel what you feel. Going through treatments for cancer is obviously a difficult time, and it is natural to feel fear, anguish, and uncertainty. It's OK to have a good cry when you feel the need. Be kind to yourself, allow people to help you during this time, and take advantage of the many things it's possible for you to do to boost your spirits on a bad day.

SUNSHINE AND FRESH AIR

Getting out in the sunshine and enjoying fresh air can be a real boost to your spirits. And experts agree that a small amount of sun exposure will keep blood levels of Vitamin D adequate. For those with fair skin, a seven-to-10-minute walk outside with arms or legs uncovered in summertime should give you the Vitamin D you need – although it's not recommended going out in the midday sun. In winter, longer sun exposure is necessary to gain any benefit.

Vitamin D is also available in foods such as liver, eggs, full-fat and soy milk, and fatty fish such as mackerel, herring, and salmon. Ask your doctor to prescribe you a free supplement if there is any concern that you may be deficient in this vitamin.

Enjoy walks on the beach or in a local park. Plant herbs and flowers in your garden, watch them grow and then appreciate their benefits. There is much to be recommended in getting in touch with nature, appreciating the seasons, seeing the magic in rainbows, and watching a sunset or sunrise.

NUTRITION

There are so many wonderful foods to eat that will improve your health and emotional wellbeing during this battle. You can actually empower yourself through what you eat.

Expensive supplements that claim miraculous results are not worth your time or money. And be suspicious of fad diets and those that exclude whole food groups or are very rigid in their approach. Delicious real food bursting with nutrition is the way to go.

Wendy Hamilton, from Optimum Health and Nutrition, has some excellent suggestions about the best foods to include in your diet – she says that the best food is that which not only looks appealing but is also good for you. Eat seasonally, and by all means choose organic food, but most importantly make sure you enjoy your food.

'Colourful vegetables and fruit can only be good for you. Health experts agree that vegetables are good for you, so aim to have at least five serves of vegetables a day, and two serves of fruit. For fruit, they are best consumed whole, rather than juiced. Think of lots of different colours when selecting fruit and vegetables. Not only does this

make your food visually appealing, but you are more likely to get all the nutrients you need from a variety of colours.

Wendy has devised the following informative list to help you make good choices. Every food has different qualities and benefits, so think variety when eating. Here are some great foods to consider:

- Red: beetroot, red onions, red cabbage, tomatoes, red peppers (also known as capsicums)

- Orange: pumpkin, kumara, carrots, apricots (all of which are high in Vitamin A or beta carotene)

- Blue: blueberries, full of antioxidants, make a great snack or dessert and are especially delicious served with yoghurt

- Green: kale, silverbeet, bok choy, spinach, asparagus, avocado, broccoli, cauliflower, Brussels sprouts, cabbage. And don't forget green herbs: rocket, watercress, coriander, parsley, basil, chives, mint.

'Other wonder foods include the onion family – leeks for winter, onions, and garlic. Sprouts are also very good.

'Nuts and seeds are indeed wonderful foods. For seeds to grow they have to be a powerhouse of nutrients.

They are full of minerals, good oils, omega-3 and omega-6. In the case of nuts, purchase them whole rather than ground as the shell protects the contents from oxidation, and eat them raw. Beneficial nuts include almonds, macadamias, walnuts, pecans, cashews, hazelnuts and Brazil nuts while chia seeds, flaxseeds, pumpkin and sesame seeds are all powerhouses of nutrients. Have them raw not pre-roasted.

'Choose good quality oils such as extra-virgin olive oil, macadamia, coconut or avocado oil to cook with or dress salads and vegetables. Apple cider vinegar is far less acidic than many other kinds, making it a good choice. Use herbs and spices to make food taste good, eg cinnamon. As for meat, use good quality. It is much better to have small amounts of good quality meat, than to go for poor quality.'

Fermented foods are excellent for the gut advises Wendy, as a lot of the drugs used in cancer treatments whip out the good bacteria. To counteract this, she recommends sauerkraut and kimchi (a Korean form of sauerkraut with more vegetables than traditional sauerkraut).

EXERCISE

Engaging in a moderate amount of physical activity while going through cancer treatments will result in improved mood and emotional states. Exercise can promote psychological wellbeing as well as improve the quality of life. It can improve self-esteem at this time, increase energy level, and decrease symptoms associated with depression.

I talked to Lou James, a cancer rehabilitation expert from PINC & STEEL, about exercise and people's emotional wellbeing.

'There are lots of different stages that people can go through when they have had cancer, and they have to allow themselves time for healing, which can take a while. Probably the most important thing is self-compassion, which is interesting because while people tend to show compassion to someone else with cancer, they are not nearly as kind when they find themselves in this situation. They tell themselves they'll be fine and expect to go back to work and just learn to cope – so the compassion for themselves isn't there.

'We highly recommend getting expert advice on suitable exercise as it is such a beneficial activity; not just physically, but emotionally as well. Most of our treatments are one-on-one, but we now have exercise groups, not least because people get to a point where the social aspect of exercise is good, too. And because exercise is something you need to keep doing, having others around you doing it too will make it more likely you'll continue to do it. On your own you might stay motivated for a little bit, but then you'll need to be encouraged. Our exercise groups are fun, and they are also an opportunity for us to educate people about the benefits of sleeping well and good nutrition. In other words, being as well as you can after having cancer. Family members don't necessarily understand all this, but when you get together a group of people who have been through the same thing, they can provide great support for each other.'*

When people's cancer treatment comes to an end, this can be a difficult time for them emotionally as they try to pick up the pattern of their previous life. They tend to think that it's just a matter of getting on with things, which is not necessarily the case, and they may need help accordingly.

Lou is aware of the research that's been done on the emotional and psychological effects of cancer, ie the importance of maintaining independence and being able to do all the things they could do before their diagnosis. She says this needs to be addressed early, rather than waiting for the inevitable consequences to occur which can make them harder to deal with.

'When I first got involved in physio it was common for people to say to me that they did not feel normal and that they didn't know how to go back to feeling normal. By getting them physically stronger through exercise, it had a massive impact emotionally, more than I would have initially thought. And when I look at all the research that we have done since the programme began, the emotional, psychological impacts of getting fitter and stronger are massive.'

TALK IT OUT!

Talking to friends and loved ones about how you are feeling can help considerably. But sometimes this might not be enough, so consider one of the numerous counselling services available if you feel you need more help emotionally.

Your doctor can give you information about what is available in your region. Counselling can help with the shock and disbelief of diagnosis, and teach you how to manage emotions such as sadness, anger, anxiety or depression. Counselling can also help with managing emotions around appointments and learning how to talk to health professionals, so you can ask the right questions and make the best decisions. Other benefits include learning to cope with any physical changes, your sexuality, uncertainty about the future and regaining confidence – whether you are moving on from cancer treatments or facing a terminal diagnosis. This can all help with the rollercoaster of emotions you are likely to feel during this time.

PAMPERING

Don't be afraid to pamper yourself while going through cancer treatments. Indulge in a foot massage or manicure, listen to your favourite music, sit on the beach or in a park, phone a friend, treat yourself to a back or shoulder massage or a facial, enjoy a bubble bath, buy fresh flowers. These are just a few suggestions as there are so many inexpensive treats you can give yourself. Above all, do anything and everything you love to do and which will raise your spirits.

GET A PET

Pets provide wonderful solace and companionship when you are unwell, so if you don't have a pet, then consider getting one if you are an animal lover. Cats and dogs in particular can ease a patient's anxiety and elevate their mood. Through their company, they can lessen feelings of isolation that may be felt during this time and will provide a distraction to pain, stress or boredom. And research has shown that petting or snuggling with a pet can release endorphins that have a calming effect.

YOUR SPIRITUAL SIDE

Don't ignore your spiritual self. If you are comfortable about this, seek help from your local church or other inspirational faith-based organisations. Great support can be found from people who share the same faith as yourself. Many people find solace in reading the Bible and other holy texts. Your prayers and the prayers of others can uplift and carry you through the most difficult of times. Never discount a miracle!

BE ORGANISED

Before you go to any appointment or treatment, have a plan to help you get through it. You might want to take a bag of goodies and activities to keep your spirits up. Here are some suggestions by way of things to take with you:

- delicious snacks in case you get hungry

- a bottle of your favourite drink to keep you hydrated

- some light reading, maybe a feel-good novel, or a magazine to keep your mind occupied

- puzzles such as crosswords, sudoku or even a jigsaw can be relaxing

- a sketch pad and pencil, for those artistically inclined

- music is always a great option for blocking out medical procedures so plug in your headphones and relax

- a device on which you can watch a movie or TV show but keep it light and upbeat; it's not unusual for people facing cancer to avoid the daily news for a while – it's time to focus on your recovery, not the tragedies that may be unfolding around the globe

- relevant medication as you might be there for some time

- a notebook in which to write about any issues regarding your medical treatment; a great tool to refer to when you are meeting with members of your medical team

- ask a friend or family member to keep you company but avoid those with negative and depressing stories about cancer.

In short, try to do as many fun things as you have energy for when going through your treatment or waiting for an appointment. Spoil yourself whenever you can.

GET CREATIVE

Many people find keeping a journal helpful when facing cancer. Even if you have never done it before, give it a go as it may help you feel better. Start by asking yourself how you are feeling, and then pour any emotion that results onto the page. Or perhaps write a letter that you never intend to send to anyone; it can be very therapeutic to get your feelings away from your physical body and onto paper. Such a letter might even be aimed at your body and is a way to express your disappointment in what is happening. Just get those feelings onto the page and you are likely to feel better for it. This might also be a time when you try writing some poetry or a short story or even a memoir of your life!

Other people have found art can be very restorative for the soul. Whether drawing or painting on canvas, if you feel like it then do it! The idea is to create and lose yourself in the moment. This is all about the enjoyment, not the end result.

An interest in photography can also be healing. Take images of beauty wherever you find it, eg by the ocean, or perhaps a river or lake. Notice the reflection on the water. Enjoy a picnic on the grass while you're out. Photograph the clouds, the sunrise and the sunset. And don't overlook recording images of your nearest and dearest.

You might like to let other people's creativity entertain and uplift you during this time, whether it's through music, books, movies, or your favourite TV series. Draw on others' inspiration to speak to your soul and refresh it.

Lindsey Dawson, an inspirational author and public speaker, recently finished a range of treatments for cancer. Here she offers some fabulous examples of how her creativity helped her during this time, along with other valuable advice.

'I kept on working on assignments for an online art therapy diploma, which was a good distraction, and I also had an art project set up more or less permanently on my dining table which I would sit down to work at often. Getting out paints and brushes was very therapeutic. And because I had a novel in production, working on the many necessary details to make that happen served to remind me that there was a world to return to once my treatment was over.

'I also took myself off for various therapies –

such as a memorably good facial, plus head massage. This was so nice as I'd recently gone bald and my head felt like it needed some loving care. I also had a series of sessions with an energy healer who tucked crystals around me as I lay on his massage table and washed the room (and me) with the resonant sounds of crystal-bowl toning. I had several crystal-bowl sessions with two practitioners, in fact – it sounds odd, but it's hugely relaxing. And I took myself off into meditation, which is always very clearing and refreshing. There was an extraordinary miri miri massage, too (a form of traditional Maori healing), which was painful at the time but left me feeling very good indeed.

'In the middle of chemo I got grumpy, depressed and resentful (which I gather is a common emotional state for cancer patients) and went for a counselling session – though finding the right counsellor for you is important, I think. The one session was sufficient for me, but if you have a heap of issues to work through, then a long-term course could be beneficial.

'In terms of emotional coping, I tended to avoid social gatherings where I knew there'd be a lot of trivial chatter and shrieky laughing. Mostly, I wanted quiet and just couldn't take silly conversations with

people who had few cares except for what was happening for them at that moment. Shopping malls were a big switch-off, too – so much noise and commotion! Negotiating places like that wore me out. On the other hand, you don't want to be a hermit either – becoming so withdrawn from the world that you become a ghost of your former busy self.

'The trick is to take a medium path, keeping as busy as you want or need to be. And it's good to spend time with your nearest and dearest so that you keep in touch socially without getting exhausted, but can also excuse yourself if you want to without hurting anyone's feelings. It's good, for your own sake, to learn to say no more often.

'Mentally, you need to recognise you have had a huge shock. There you were sailing along, one day pretty much the same as the next, and then suddenly someone told you that you have a life-threatening illness. Even if your long-term prognosis is good and you are progressing well, I suspect that few of us who've had a cancer diagnosis ever get over being watchful and cautious. A shock does that to you – at the least it leaves lasting tender spots on your psyche and may even change your life, possibly making you rethink your whole

life and purpose and how you want to spend the rest of your days.

'Overall, be gentle with yourself. This is a huge thing you're going through.'

SOCIAL MEDIA

In researching this particular topic I reached out to Amber Arkell whose inspirational blog on Facebook, *whenthingswenttitsup*, is about facing cancer. It's an excellent example of the positive use of social media while dealing with this diagnosis.

'I started my blog as a way of keeping my friends and family up-to-date, instead of having 20 different conversations in the background. I wanted personally to inspire, educate and motivate – and my lifelong dream is to be a motivational speaker one day. So I did a video explaining my situation of being diagnosed with cancer, and that I had chemo coming, and overnight I had 700 people following my blog.

'I talked with my sister and my mum about coming up with a creative, but light-hearted name for the blog. I also wanted my blog to be honest and to not make it to be something it's not. People related to that. And once I hit around 1000 people, and kept getting good feedback I thought I should keep with it.

'I'm naturally a positive person. People have asked how I can stay so positive, but I do have down days. I keep my posts as positive as possible, but fact-based, so it's an informative process, not so much about my feelings and emotions.'

Amber's top tips for using social media while going through cancer treatments follow.

'The first thing is to decide if you want to post on a public or private forum. For me, it was about inspiring and educating other people as I went through the journey. But for other people, it might be a place where they can vent, so they are best to do this privately and keep their friends and family up-to-date – and get that social media support that they are looking for in this way. Keep the content real, and be yourself. Keep to the points you are trying to communicate, rather than waffling. You may not feel like responding to all the comments that you get, and that's OK. A collective message to people is just fine.

'If you are like me and you want to use social media to educate and inspire, then I feel a public forum is beneficial. It comes down to the individual regarding what you are comfortable with. But if you are posting on a public forum, there are things that you may choose not to share; for me these include personal matters that I have talked about with close friends. And I may never share them as they are very personal.

'You also should be aware that if you share your story on a public forum, you will get people contacting you with their stories, so you need to be prepared for that. But as I've got better and stronger and more knowledgeable about what I'm going through, hearing other peoople's stories doesn't upset me as much, although to begin with this was difficult.

'Social media isn't perfect, however. It doesn't change the fact that you are the one going through this, and some days are tough. I have had days when it is hard to see everyone's lives on social media because it looks like people are having so much fun, especially the days when I'm at home in bed because of chemo. But there is also so much that is positive. My blog has brought women together, so it is very much about going beyond myself. And by communicating online, some women have gone on to meet each other in person, so real friendships have been formed.'

LOOKING FORWARD

If you have a good prognosis, it can be helpful to look forward to your life after you have completed treatment. Some people like to plan a holiday (discuss optimal timing with your doctor), while others like to ease back into pursuits and interests they enjoyed before.

It's not uncommon to find yourself hard hit emotionally after completing your treatments, so don't feel alarmed if this happens to you. If you are feeling depressed, do go and seek help. Some people see a counsellor at this stage, but above all be kind to yourself as you ease back into 'regular' life.

Be aware that your physical and emotional healing won't take a linear path, but will probably be a case of two steps forward and one step back, not least because recovery from cancer treatments can often take longer than the treatments themselves. Remember to take things easy in your early stages of recovery. And because we are all individual, there is no one pathway that will take you into the future, though support is key as you begin to return to your normal life.

Many things can't be controlled in life, and having cancer – along with any ongoing effects or consequences of surgeries and treatments – is one of

them. However there is much you can control – your attitude to life, the things you choose to do from this moment on, and the people you surround yourself with. Initially you may need to think outside the box so it doesn't become too much for you to manage, eg if you are eager to get back to your work perhaps you can work some of the time from home. And if you are keen to go travelling, work on an itinerary that is fun, but also practical; that will take into account that you might not have a full tank of energy for some time.

Above all, step into the future with hope and confidence. Face any fear you have about the cancer returning head on, and then set it aside. Delight in your life now you are through your battle. Value it, listen to your intuition and know you are so much more than just a body. Follow your passions, surround yourself with quality people and nurture your precious self in body, soul, and spirit.

BAKING

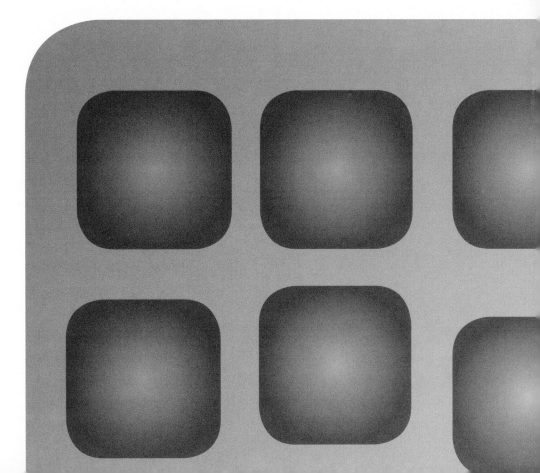

Clafoutis

4–6   PREP: 10 min   COOKING TIME: 40 min

INGREDIENTS:

1 tbsp **butter**

110g (3.9oz) **sugar**

6 **eggs**

1 tsp **vanilla extract**

110g (3.9oz) **flour**

650g (23oz) **berries**, eg blackberries, cherries, blueberries

icing sugar, to dust

Preheat the oven to 230°C.

Grease a ceramic baking dish with the butter and scatter a pinch of the sugar over the top.

Break the eggs into a large mixing bowl and whisk together. Beat in the sugar well so that everything is fully combined. Add the vanilla extract. Sift in the flour and fold it into the mixture so that it is only just incorporated (ie resist the temptation to overwork the mixture). Pour the batter into the prepared baking dish and scatter the berries over the top. Bake in the oven for 35–40 minutes or until the top is a beautiful golden brown. Test to see if it is done by inserting a skewer into the centre; it should come out clean. Dust some icing sugar over the top, and serve.

Sam: If you do use frozen berries, don't defrost them beforehand, as they will go soggy and disintegrate; instead, just put them into the batter frozen. Don't feel that you have to stick with berries, either. Canned peaches, drained, are lovely. You may want to fold some melted chocolate into the batter, perhaps adding some chopped pear as well before popping in the oven. Give this recipe a go with plums, apple, grapes and so on. I like to serve it with good ice cream, or maybe some runny cream.

Karen: Berries are high in antioxidants so choose the berries you enjoy most and feel justifiably self-righteous about what you are eating!

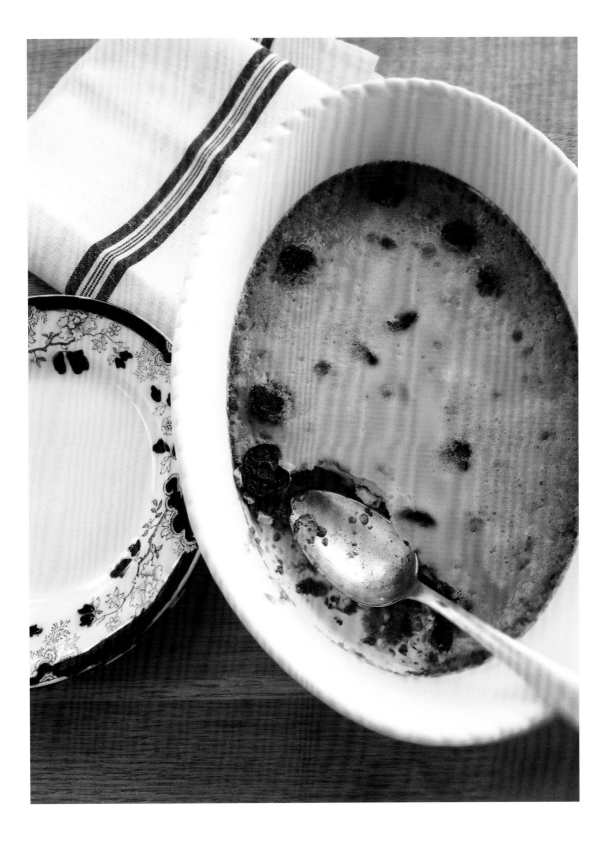

Banana, Chocolate and Almond Cake

◯ 6–8   PREP: 15 min   COOKING TIME: 55 min

INGREDIENTS:

150ml **vegetable oil**

200g (7oz) **brown sugar**

1 tsp **vanilla essence**

2 **eggs**

350g (12.3oz) **ripe bananas**, roughly mashed

70g (2.4oz) **Greek-style yoghurt**

50g (1.7oz) **roast almonds**, roughly chopped

150g (5.3oz) **chocolate**, roughly chopped

1 tsp **baking soda**

1 tsp **baking powder**

1 tsp **cinnamon**

pinch of **salt**

220g (7.7oz) **wholemeal flour**

Preheat the oven to 170°C.

Grease a regular loaf tin (mine is 26x11cm) and line with baking paper.

In a large mixing bowl, beat together the vegetable oil, brown sugar, vanilla essence and eggs.

Add the mashed banana and yoghurt, followed by the almonds and chocolate, and mix well to combine. Combine the baking soda, baking powder, cinnamon, salt and flour in another bowl, then sift the dry mixture into the banana mixture and gently fold in so that everything is only just incorporated. Transfer the mixture to the lined tin and smooth off the top. Bake in the preheated oven for 45–55 minutes or until a skewer inserted into the centre comes out clean. Allow the cake to cool down in the tin before turning it out and polishing it off.

Sam: Loaf cakes seem to stand somewhere in the middle between health-conscious treat and all-out guilty pleasure. This is indeed a bit of both. Use whatever type of chocolate you like.

Karen: Sam is right when he talks about the health benefits of this loaf, which is packed with fibre and vitamins. And how wonderful that it is also so yummy.

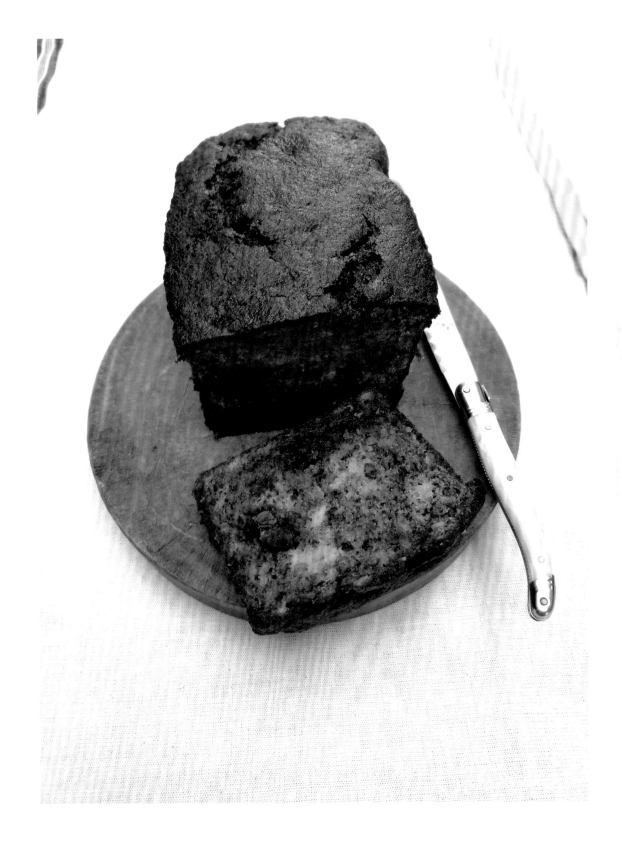

Pear and Walnut Gingerbread

4–6   PREP: 20 min   COOKING TIME: 45 min

INGREDIENTS:

60g (2.1oz) **butter**

100g (3.5oz) **brown sugar**

3 **pears**, peeled, quartered and cored

handful of **walnuts**

60g (2.1oz) **butter**

125g (3.5oz) **brown sugar**

2 tbsp **treacle** or **golden syrup**

1 **egg**

½ cup (125ml) **milk**

125g (4.4oz) **flour**

½ tsp **baking powder**

¼ tsp **salt**

2 tsp **cinnamon**

1 tsp **ginger**

¼ tsp **nutmeg**

pinch of **ground cloves**

Preheat the oven to 180°C. Line a round cake tin with baking paper.

Melt the first lot of butter and brown sugar in a small saucepan. Pour over the bottom of the cake tin and spread all over to cover the base.

Arrange the quartered pears and the walnuts over the top of the butter and sugar mixture.

In a large bowl beat the second lot of butter and brown sugar together until light and fluffy. Mix in the treacle or golden syrup, followed by the egg, followed by the milk. Sift in the remaining ingredients and fold them in until the mixture is combined. Pour the batter into the tin and over the top of the pears, then smooth off the surface.

Bake for 45 minutes in the preheated oven. Then remove the gingerbread from the oven and allow it to cool in the tin. Place a plate face side down over the tin and turn everything carefully over so that the cake slides out onto the plate. Peel off the baking paper and serve.

Sam: My grandmother makes the best gingerbread in the world. Obviously I'm being totally unbiased. Many people will attest to Esther's legendary gingerbread, and to avoid a fight with several well-known food personalities, I'll say it's nearly first equal. Gingerbread and pear is a superb combo, especially in autumn when pears are lovely and crisp. Beurre bosc or Doyenne de Comice will both work well in this recipe. Serve warm with one of the usual suspects; ice cream, or yoghurt.

Karen: Ginger and pear are a great health combo full of dietary fibre, antioxidants, minerals and vitamins. And, of course, ginger is great for settling a dodgy tummy.

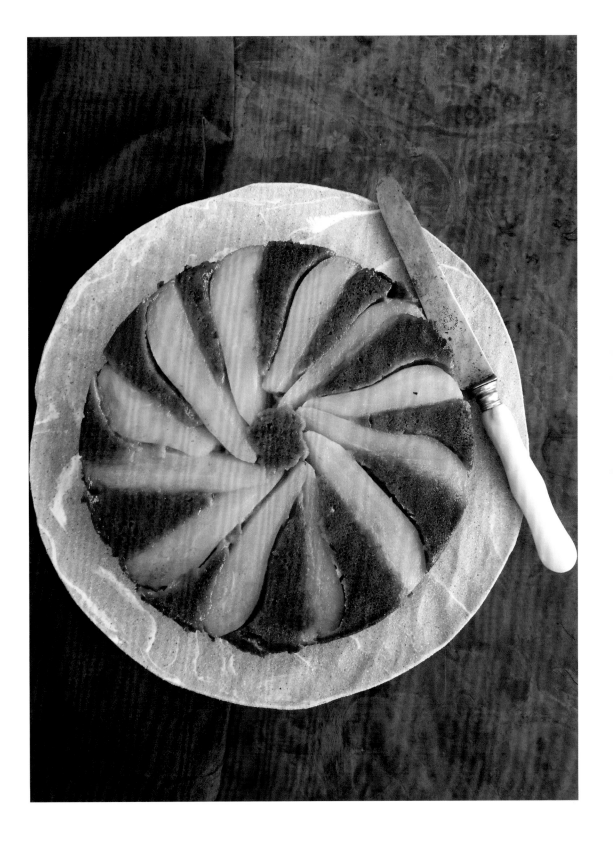

Tarte Tatin

4–6   PREP: 10 min   COOKING TIME: 30 min

INGREDIENTS:

3 large apples or golden peaches

400g (14oz) puff pastry

200g (7oz) brown sugar

220g (7.7oz) butter

Preheat the oven to 200°C.

Peel, halve and core the apples, then cut each half into four (if you are using peaches, remove the stones and do the same).

Take a large oven-proof frying pan (I used a 30cm one). Roll out the pastry on a floured surface to a thickness of about 5cm. Cut it into a round slightly bigger than the circumference of the pan.

Place the pan over a medium-high heat. Add the butter and brown sugar and let it bubble up for several minutes, taking care not to let it burn. Arrange the apple slices neatly around the bottom of the pan, packing them in so that the entire surface is covered. Let the caramel bubble away for a little longer, then carefully cover the apples with the puff pastry, tucking the edges into the sides of the pan.

Place the pan into the preheated oven and bake for 25–30 minutes until the pastry is puffed and golden brown. Leave to cool down for several minutes, then run a knife all the way around the edge of the pastry to loosen it. Place a large plate or serving dish over the top and carefully invert the tart upside down, with the help of several tea towels. Word of warning: when inverting, be extremely wary of any rogue runny caramel as it will burn like lava (I have the scars to prove it).

Serve immediately.

Sam: This classic dessert has been an institution since the Tatin sisters made the apparent accident of putting pastry over the top of caramelised apples and banging them in the oven in the hope of saving what was meant to be an apple pie.

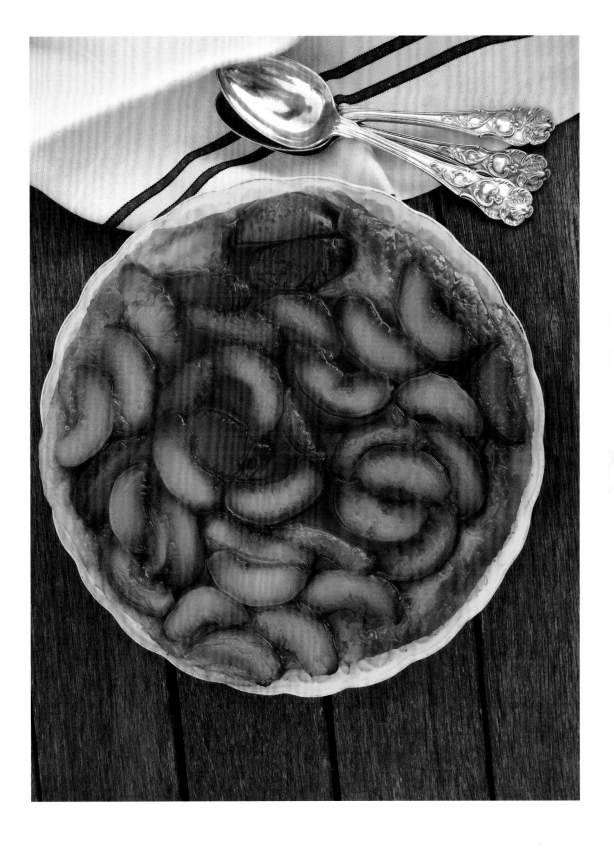

Carrot Cake

8–10   PREP: 25 min   COOKING TIME: 50 min

CAKE:

1½ cups (375ml) **light oil**

480g (16.9oz) **brown sugar**

4 **eggs**

1 tsp **vanilla essence**

zest of 1 **orange**

280g (9.8z) **wholemeal flour**

1½ tsp **cinnamon**

1 tsp **salt**

about 3 cups **grated carrot**

120g (4.2oz) **chopped walnuts**

2 tsp **baking soda**

ICING:

200g (7oz) **cream cheese**

120g (4.2oz) **icing sugar**

60g (2.1oz) **melted butter**

1 tsp **vanilla**

zest of 1 **orange**

Preheat the oven to 160°C.

Line a round collapsible cake tin with baking paper.

In a large mixing bowl combine the oil and sugar. Beat in the eggs, one by one, followed by the vanilla and orange zest and mix well. Stir in the flour, cinnamon and salt, and fold in the carrot and walnuts and incorporate into the mixture. Finally, add the baking soda and quickly stir in well. Pour the mixture into the lined tin and bake in the preheated oven for about 50 minutes, until a skewer or knife poked into the middle comes out clean. Remove from the oven and let it cool down completely – just leave it in the tin.

Once it is completely cool, remove the cake from the tin and transfer carefully to a plate. Combine all of the five icing ingredients and beat together well. Spoon the icing onto the cooled cake. I think that a good inch of icing on top of the cake is essential. Trust me on this. It is that delicious. This will keep well for several days, but I know from experience that it won't last that long anyway.

Sam: There are plenty of perfectly adequate carrot cake recipes out there. Of course I'm going to tell you that this is the best of the lot. It is my mother's recipe and that woman knows her stuff. This is something completely different. I'm not one for using the word 'moist' when I can help it, but when placed alongside more tolerable words like flavourful, rich, dense, and, well, frankly delicious, you have this cake in a nutshell.

Karen: Tasty and packed with fibre, vitamins and minerals, this is a fabulous carrot cake.

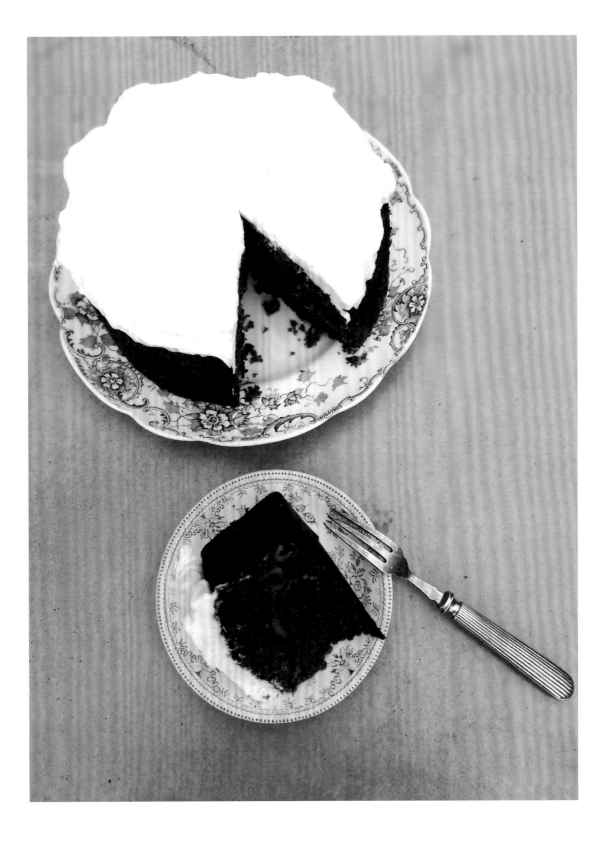

Pear and Chocolate Crumble

6–8   PREP: 25 min   COOKING TIME: 30 min

INGREDIENTS:

5 **pears**, peeled, quartered lengthways and cored

zest and **juice** of 1 **lemon**

1 tsp **vanilla essence** or ½ tsp **vanilla paste**

175g (6.2oz) **brown sugar**

100g (3.5oz) **dark chocolate**, roughly chopped

100g (3.5oz) **butter**

200g (7oz) **flour**

100g (3.5oz) **oats**

Preheat the oven to 180°C.

In a saucepan over a medium heat combine the pears with the lemon zest and juice, vanilla essence/paste, 100ml water and 100g of the brown sugar. Allow the sugar to dissolve into the water and become slightly caramelised before removing from the heat. Transfer the mixture to a large ovenproof dish and scatter the chopped chocolate over the top of the pears.

In a food processor whizz the butter, flour and remaining sugar together so that it resembles breadcrumbs. Turn out into a bowl and using your hands rub the oats into the mixture. Scatter over the pear mixture and bake in the oven for about 25–30 minutes until the top is nicely golden brown.

Sam: Make sure you choose a good dark chocolate to offset the sweetness of this dish. Serve with runny cream, custard, ice cream, or all three.

Karen: The dark chocolate really makes this fabulous crumble; although it's a sprinkle of decadence, it offers many anti-oxidants and other health benefits.

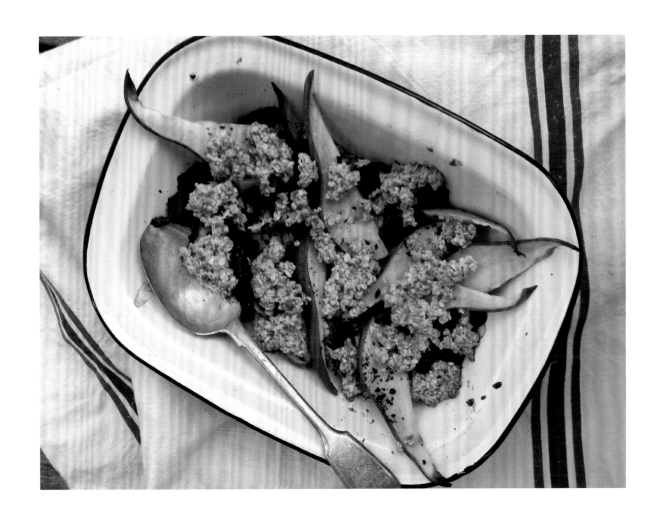

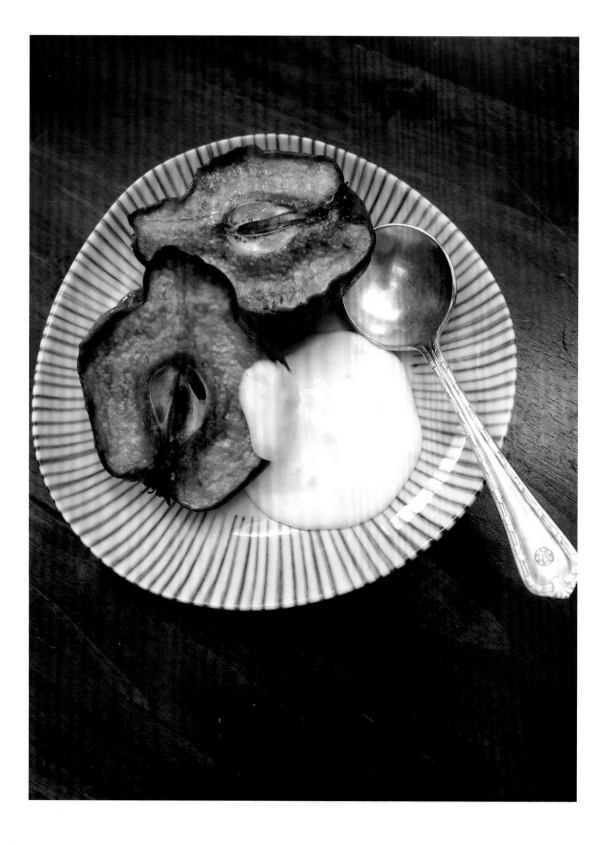

Baked Quinces with Lemon Mascarpone

 6   PREP: 10 min   COOKING TIME: 30 min   GF

INGREDIENTS:

3 **quinces**, halved

2 **cinnamon sticks**

1 **lemon**

100g (3.5oz) **brown sugar**

1 tbsp **butter**

150g (5.3oz) **mascarpone**

zest and **juice** of 1 **lemon**

1 tbsp **icing sugar**

Preheat the oven to 170°C.

Arrange the halved quinces and the cinnamon sticks in a roasting dish or ovenproof frying pan. Add 200ml water, then zest the lemon over the top and squeeze in the juice. Sprinkle the brown sugar over the top and dot over the butter, then put in the oven to bake for about half an hour, until the quinces are soft and have turned a delicate pinky colour, and the liquid has reduced to a lovely sticky sort of sauce.

Remove from the oven and allow them to cool down a little.

In the meantime, whip together the mascarpone, lemon zest and juice, and icing sugar until smooth to serve alongside the quinces.

Sam: Autumn is a great time for making simple desserts like this, which also serve as a terrific accompaniment to porridge or bircher with a bit of yoghurt and honey. Some good vanilla ice-cream is a pretty fantastic alternative to the mascarpone.

Karen: Quince is a good source of Vitamin C, zinc, iron and dietary fibre. Enjoy!

Caramel and Almond Slice

10–15   PREP: 20 min   COOKING TIME: 40 min

BASE:

200g (7 oz) **soft butter**

220g (7.7 oz) **castor sugar**

zest and **juice** of 1 **lemon**

1 tsp **vanilla essence**

350g (12.3oz) **flour**

1 tsp **baking powder**

TOPPING:

150g (5.3 oz) **butter**

1 tbsp **golden syrup**

1 x 395g (13.9 oz) can **condensed milk**

zest and **juice** of 1 **lemon**

½ cup (60g/2.1oz) of **flaked almonds**

Preheat the oven to 180°C.

Grease and line a slice tin (mine is 32x20cm) with baking paper.

Make the topping first. In a bain-marie (a bowl over a pan of gently simmering water) melt all the topping ingredients together except for the flaked almonds until you have a smooth, consistent mixture. Take it off the heat and let it cool down a bit.

While the topping cools a little, make the base. Beat together the butter, castor sugar, lemon zest and juice in mixer until light and fluffy. Sift in the flour and baking powder and fold them in to create a soft dough.

Press the mixture into the lined tin, then carefully pour the topping mixture evenly over the base and smooth it off. Sprinkle the almonds over the top, pop in the oven and then bake for about 40 minutes. Take care not to let it get too brown on top. Allow to cool completely before cutting.

This will last for up to a week in an airtight tin.

Sam: I have a fascination with small town bakeries. This recipe is based on one we used at the Dunsandel Store. Upon opening, our friend Nicola Groundwater came to the rescue with a big wad of wonderful old baking recipes, and this was a lasting favourite.

Karen: The beauty of Sam's wonderful baking recipes is that as they are all cooked from scratch you know exactly what is in them, ie no nasty additives and preservatives.

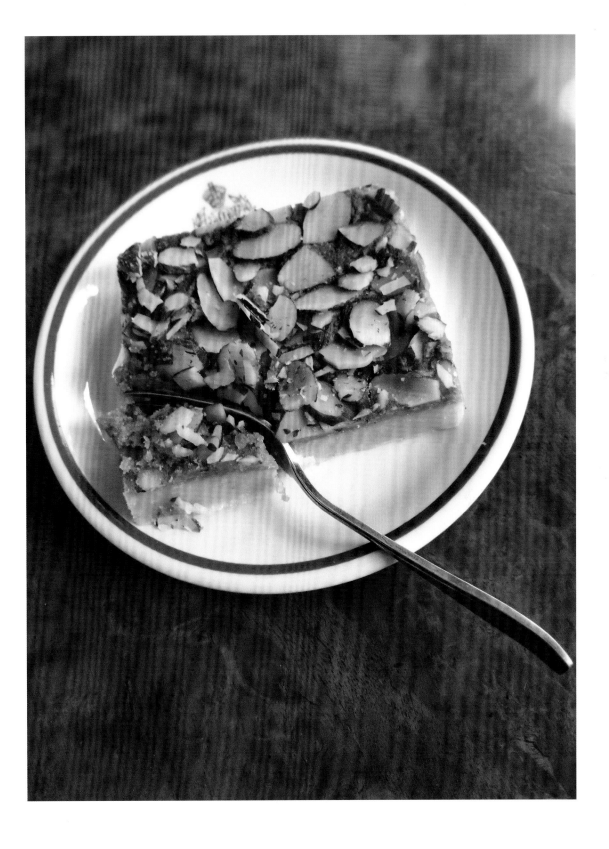

Chocolate and Almond Brownie

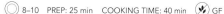 8–10   PREP: 25 min   COOKING TIME: 40 min   GF

BROWNIE:

200g (7oz) **dark chocolate**

4 tbsp **strong coffee**

150g (5.3 oz) **castor sugar**

150g (5.3 oz) **butter**

125g (4.4 oz) **ground almonds**

5 **eggs**, separated

CHOCOLATE GANACHE:

60ml **cream**

1 tbsp **butter**

110g **good quality chocolate**

30ml **coffee**

Preheat the oven to 180°C.

Grease and line a 20x20cm square tin with baking paper.

Melt the chocolate, coffee, sugar and butter in a heavy saucepan over a low heat, stirring well to combine. When everything has melted together, add the ground almonds and beat in the egg yolks one by one. Take off the heat and allow the mixture to cool.

Beat the egg whites until stiff peaks form. Stir 3 tablespoons of egg white into the chocolate mix, then gently fold in the rest of the egg white.

Pour the mixture into the prepared tin and bake for about 40 minutes or until a skewer comes out only just clean (don't overcook it!). Remove from the oven and leave to cool in the tin (note: the middle will drop slightly, so don't panic when it does).

Allow to cool completely before icing and cutting into squares.

To make the icing, with a rich, coffee-laced chocolate ganache: bring the cream and butter almost to the boil, then pour them over the top of the chocolate and coffee. Leave to stand for several minutes, then stir gently to combine everything into a smooth icing. Use to ice the brownies before serving.

Sam: Don't overcook this, as it will end up all horrible and dry, and quite underwhelming. Ice if you like – I still haven't decided whether it is nicer with or without! Best served with a bit of cream and perhaps some poached berries to cut the sweetness.

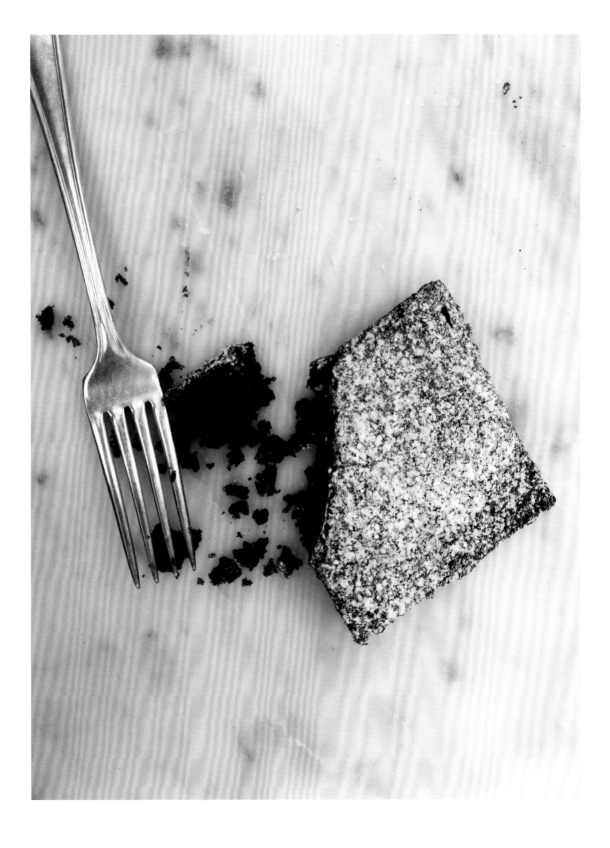

Coconut Tapioca with Mango, Lime and Passionfruit

6–8   PREP: 20 min   COOKING TIME: 30 min   GF   DF

INGREDIENTS:

150g (5.3oz) small **pearl tapioca**

1 **vanilla pod**

250ml (7oz) **coconut cream**

200g (7oz) **sugar**

2 **eggs**

2 **mangoes**, peeled and chopped

zest and **juice** of 1 **lime**

1 fresh **passionfruit** or 1 tbsp **passionfruit pulp**

In a saucepan combine the tapioca, 500ml water and the vanilla pod. Gently heat to a simmer over a low heat, stirring occasionally, until the tapioca is tender and translucent and the water has been absorbed.

Remove the pan from the heat and stir in the coconut cream. Set aside and leave to cool down.

In a large bowl, whisk together the sugar and eggs. Gradually whisk in a third of the cooled tapioca mixture, then combine with the remaining mix.

Return the mixture to the pan and cook over a low heat for several minutes to allow it to thicken. Remove the vanilla bean, scrape out the seeds and add to the mixture. Take off the heat and set aside to cool.

Mix the chopped mango with the lime juice and zest and the pulp from the passionfruit. Layer the fruit mixture in glasses alternating it with the cooled tapioca mixture.

Sam: I can proudly say that I have converted plenty of committed tapioca haters with this dessert. Canned mango is absolutely fine, by the way. Similarly, you can use sweet passionfruit pulp, but fresh is always better.

Karen: Passionfruit is full of Vitamin C, which is great for your overall health.

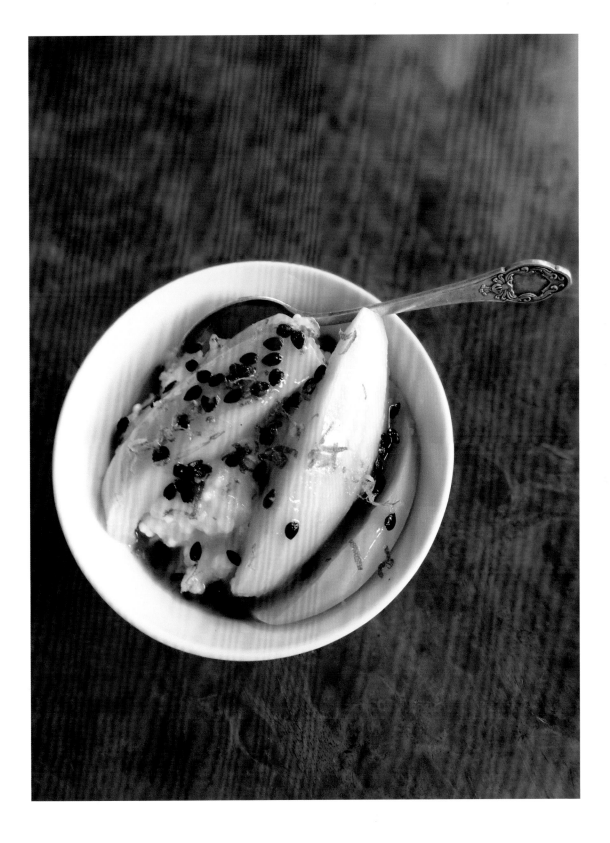

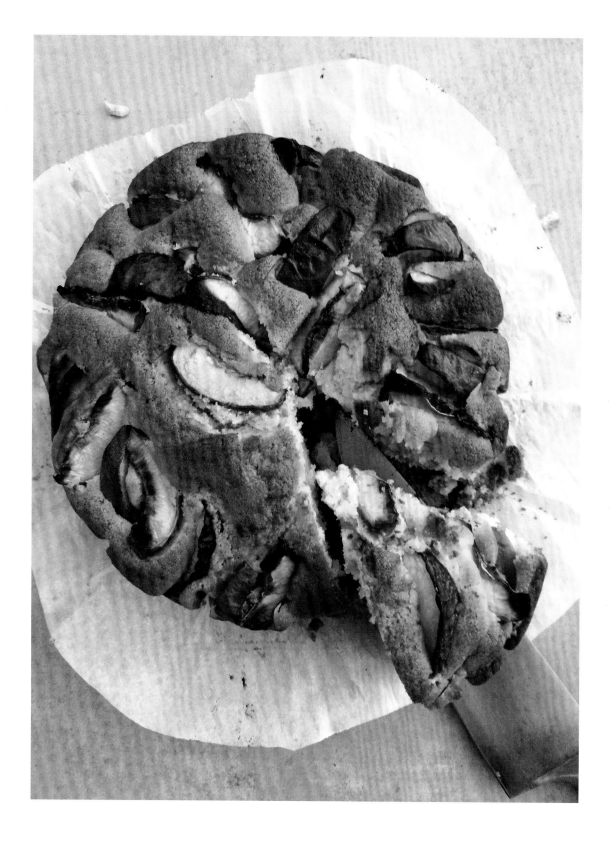

A Damn Good Nectarine Cake

8–10   PREP: 20 min   COOKING TIME: 60 min

INGREDIENTS:

5 large **ripe nectarines**

320g (11.3oz) **butter**

300g (10.5oz) **sugar**

3 **eggs**

250ml **milk**

zest and **juice** of 2 **lemons**

400g (14.1oz) **self-raising flour**

1½ tsp **baking powder**

Preheat the oven to 180°C.

Line a large 20 cm round cake tin with baking paper. Slice the nectarines and discard the stones.

In a large bowl beat the butter and sugar together in usual fashion until light and fluffy. Beat in the eggs, followed by the milk and the lemon zest and juice. Sift in the flour and baking powder and fold it into the mixture.

Pour the mixture into the lined tin. Spread the nectarines slices over the top, sprinkle with a little more sugar and bake for approximately 1 hour or until a skewer inserted into the centre tells you that it has only just set.

Allow the cake to cool before dusting with icing sugar and devouring with whipped cream or ice cream for dessert.

Sam: This cake is inspired by the extraordinary Gretta Anna, an Australasian food icon who doesn't get a fraction of the kudos that she deserves. You can use virtually any fresh stone fruit that takes your fancy: Peaches, plums, cherries and even apples with a bit of cinnamon are particularly delicious alternatives.

Karen: The nectarines, or other fresh stone fruit you might use in this tasty cake, are a great way to include extra vitamins and minerals in your diet.

Apple, Hazelnut and Caramel Pinwheel Scones

8–10   PREP: 25 min   COOKING TIME: 20–25 min

INGREDIENTS:

120g (4.2oz) **butter**

100g (3.5oz) **brown sugar**

2 **apples**, thinly sliced

500g (17.6oz) **self-raising flour**

2 tsp **baking powder**

zest of 1 **lemon**

100g (3.5 oz) **cold butter**

300ml **milk**

½ cup (125g/4.4oz) **hazelnuts**, roasted and roughly chopped

Preheat the oven to 200°C.

In a saucepan over a low heat, melt together the butter and brown sugar and let it bubble and cook for about 3 minutes so that you have a runny caramel sauce. Remove from the heat, add the apples and toss to coat. Set aside for a minute to cool down while you make the scone dough.

In a bowl combine the flour and baking powder. Mix in the lemon zest, then grate in the butter and rub it into the flour mix. Make a well in the middle and add the milk. Gently mix everything together so that it is just combined into a soft dough. Do not over-mix.

On a floured surface, roll the dough out into a rectangle of about 25x40cm, and to a thickness of about 0.5cm. Spread the apple mixture evenly over the top of the dough, and retain any leftover sauce for glazing once the pinwheels have been cooked. Sprinkle the chopped hazelnuts over the top of the sliced apple. Carefully roll up the dough lengthways into a log, then cut into 2–3cm pieces. Arrange the scones on a lined baking tray.

Bake for about 20–25 minutes until the scones have risen and turned golden. Use the leftover caramel to drizzle over the top of the baked scones.

Sam: I like a bit of lemon zest in the dough to offset the sweetness. Roasting the hazelnuts beforehand will bring out the flavour wonderfully. When baked in a round, cast iron pan, arranged in a circular pattern, these look pretty appealing.

Karen: Hazelnuts are good sources of calcium, Vitamin E and Vitamin B. Vitamin E is really good for maintaining healthy skin, hair and nails.

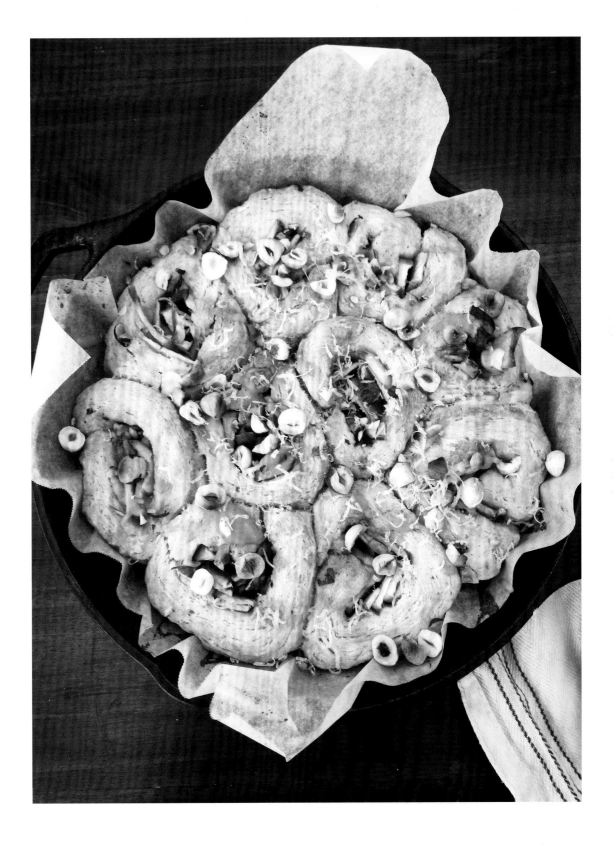

Sam's Cheese Scones

makes 8–10 scones   PREP: 5 min   COOKING TIME: 15 min

INGREDIENTS:

2 cups (500g, 17.5oz) **self-raising flour**

1 tsp **baking powder**

½ tsp **salt**

pinch of **cayenne pepper**

100g (3.5oz) **cold butter**

75g (2.6oz) **cheddar**, grated

75g (2.6oz) **parmesan**, grated

handful of **flat leaf parsley**, finely chopped

1 cup (250ml/8.8oz) **milk**

1 **egg**, beaten

Preheat the oven to 200°C.

Into a large mixing bowl sift together the flour, baking powder, salt and cayenne pepper. Grate in the cold butter and rub through the dry ingredients. Add both cheeses and the parsley and combine well. Create a well in the centre of the mixture. Pour in the milk and bring in the dry ingredients gently, combining everything until you have a soft, consistent dough (take care not to overwork the dough). Roll out the dough to a thickness of between 3 and 4cm, then use a cutter to cut into rounds or squares. Transfer the scones to a lined baking tray and brush with beaten egg.

Bake for 5 minutes at 200°C, then reduce the temperature down to 180°C and bake for another 8–10 minutes until the scones are well risen and golden brown. Remove from the oven and allow them to cool a little for 5 minutes before serving with lashings of good quality butter.

Sam: Scones don't really need the effort that people often think they do. In fact, the less effort, the better. Don't overwork the dough; you are merely combining the ingredients. Use leftover pieces of cheese in the fridge, the stronger the better. For a sweet counterpart, omit the cheese, parsley and cayenne, and add instead ¼ cup of sugar, ½ cup of chopped dates and the zest of a lemon.

Karen: Delicious, light and tasty; these are really easy to prepare and make good filling food suitable for the entire family. As a bonus, cheese is a great source of protein, calcium, Vitamin A and Vitamin B12.

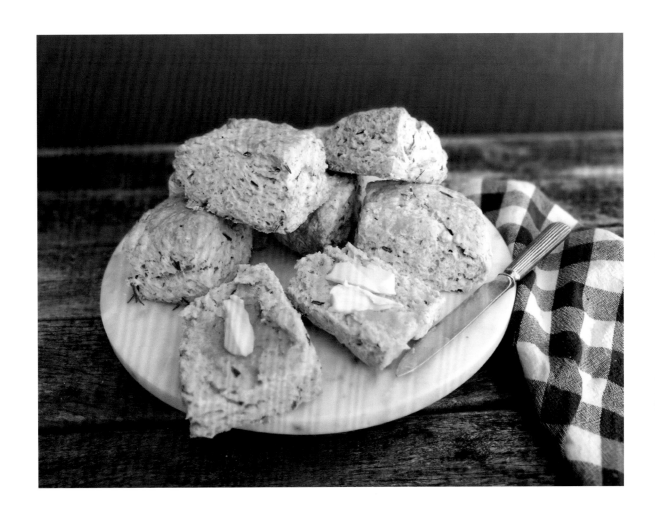

Rice Pudding with Stone Fruit

4–6   PREP: 10 min   COOKING TIME: 120 min   GF

INGREDIENTS:

5 tbsp **short-grain white rice**

3 tbsp **golden castor sugar**

3 cups (750ml) **milk**

½ tsp **vanilla extract**

2 tsp **butter**

2 **nectarines**, **plums** or **peaches**, thinly sliced and stones removed

Preheat the oven to 150°C on bake function.

In a ceramic baking dish combine the rice, sugar, milk and vanilla extract. Dot small pieces of the butter over the mixture and scatter the sliced fruit over the top. Bake for 2 hours, stirring occasionally, until the rice is creamy and cooked. Allow to cool for 5 minutes or so before serving.

Sam: *This is one of my favourite desserts of all time. Despite the cooking time, it is ridiculously easy to make, and you can use whatever fruit you like (or not use fruit at all; a grating of fresh nutmeg sometimes is enough).*

Karen: *Fruits like nectarines, plums and peaches are full of Vitamin C and are also a great source of fibre.*

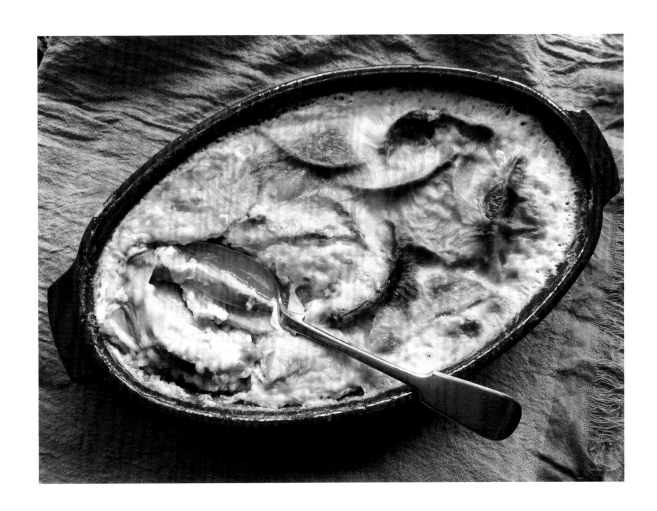

Bircher

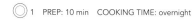

1   PREP: 10 min   COOKING TIME: overnight

INGREDIENTS:

1 cup (90g/3.2oz) **oats**

orange juice

1 **apple** or **pear**

other options listed in recipe

Before you go to bed, soak the oats. Depending on how many you want to serve the next day, add enough oats (I think a cup per person is fine) to a large bowl and then pour in enough good orange juice to cover them by about 1cm. Cover and leave to soak overnight in the fridge.

In the morning, grate in some apple or pear; the more the better. Finely chop up some banana if you like. It is a brilliant way of using up frozen berries, since the juice will run through everything, but that being said, nothing compares with fresh berries. When they are in season, I like to use fresh strawberries quartered lengthways, blueberries and boysenberries. Poor wee raspberries seem to disintegrate in an instant.

If a bit of extra sweetness is your thing, melt some good quality honey, be it manuka, clover or whatever takes your fancy, in the microwave or gently in a saucepan and then stir into the mix.

Other additions could include long desiccated coconut threads, lemon zest and juice, a good dollop of yoghurt or coconut cream, flax seeds, pumpkin seeds, roasted almonds, walnuts and hazelnuts. Chop and change as you see fit.

Sam: Muesli is a diminutive variation of the Swiss-German word 'mues', meaning to mash, and it was pioneered by Swiss doctor Maximilian Bircher-Benner (sounds like a character from a Monty Python sketch) for his patients.

Karen: Bircher is a great way to start the day as oats are packed with fibre and anti-oxidants.

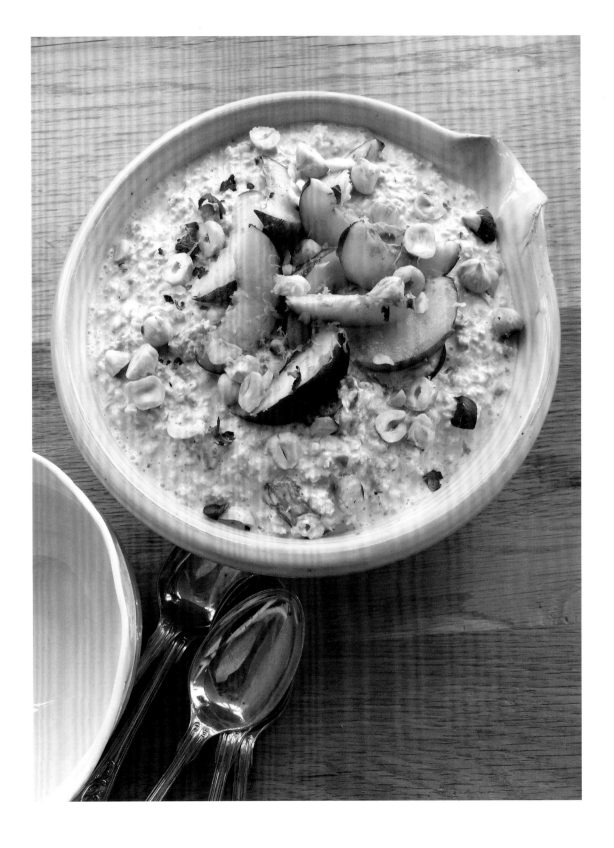

Children

PRACTICAL IDEAS FOR PARENTS

'It was awful how sick he got. It's hard to watch your kid go through that and not be able to do anything for them. And he is looking at you thinking, "Why are you doing this to me?"'
— Susan

'It was distressing to see my daughter go through the treatments, but at the same time I could only admire her resilience and the way she bounced back each time.' — Olivia

For parents of a child going through cancer treatments, this is a hugely challenging time and a daunting task indeed. Chelsea Prout, a children's cancer nurse, and a caring professional working at the coalface of cancer in young ones, gave me some practical tips that may help families during this difficult time.

EXHAUSTION

Exhaustion is something that affects cancer patients of any age, but in the case of children it is obviously something that parents get concerned about. Chelsea advises them to try not to worry about it too much and instead take things day by day.

'Children bounce back, even though they can go downhill very quickly. But equally they can soon return to normal. So you just have to take those moments when they are feeling really good, when they want to do things they didn't want to do before. And because they live in the moment, when they are well they don't really remember being unwell.'

LACK OF APPETITE

Low appetite is common in children who have cancer. Chelsea urges parents not to obviously push their children to eat. Sometimes you just need to let them sleep or relax.

'Of course, keeping up the calories is important for energy, but at these times they are also likely to suffer from a type of exhaustion that is not linked to food, in which case there is not much you can do except allow whatever is going to happen. If your child wants to simply sit and watch TV, instead of eating, try not to stress too much about it.

'If their appetite is poor, the worst thing you can do is to present them with food they don't feel like eating, which means choosing food they will like. I recommend preparing any meals away from the child, preferably behind closed doors, to keep the cooking smells from bothering them. Serve small portions little and often and don't worry about what time they want to eat. If they snack on food at irregular times, it doesn't matter. They are still eating, which is really important.

'It's particularly important in the case of young children to make the food on the plate look attractive. Try to incorporate an element of play if you can by utilising shapes and colours in a fun way, and by choosing things they can pick up and move around while they are eating. This will make it much more appealing to them.

'Never punish a child for not eating. However, rewards can work well, especially if you treat your child with something that they would really enjoy. Don't necessarily turn off the TV when children are eating either. For some children it is a good distraction, and they will eat more without realising it while watching a favourite show. If it takes a long time for your child

to eat, that doesn't matter either. As long as the food doesn't go off, it is fine.'

As a general rule, it is best to focus on offering savoury rather than sweet food, as children more often than not go off the latter. Check out the selection of recipes designed to tempt children on page 189.

CONSTIPATION AND DIARRHOEA

Chelsea notes that increasing the fibre in your child's diet through feeding them wholefoods and lots of fruit and veges will help with constipation issues.

'Prunes are good, as well as raw veges. If necessary, incorporate them into foods so the child can't see them. Or perhaps even sprinkle them on top of foods. Basically anything with more fibre is going to help. Unfortunately, though, many of the medications they'll be taking cause this constipation, making it a common problem.'

As for diarrhoea, Chelsea says this is also very common. And it's not unusual for a child to suffer from this one day and constipation the next. It is important to keep the fluids and electrolytes and salts up and to ensure the child's diet changes to reflect what is happening. For example, if a child is on steroids they run a bit of a risk of retaining fluid, in which case adding extra salt increases the risk. Light broths and soups in this instance are a good option. Diarrhoea can cause the body to lose a lot of potassium so this is the time to eat bananas, which contain good amounts of this mineral. Increase the child's fluid intake as much as possible – and make it an attractive option for them by offering them a variety of drinks. It doesn't have to be just water. Ice blocks and lemonade, fruit juices and uncaffeinated sports drinks, are all good choices.

'It can be a little bit difficult to know if children are having problems with constipation or diarrhoea unless they are still wearing nappies. It's good to create a dialogue, especially with older kids, so everyone concerned feels comfortable discussing the subject. As a parent, you need to know exactly what is going on with them, which is easy with some children, but more difficult if they are naturally shy children. Just make sure that however you choose to discuss it that it works for the child.'

NAUSEA

Because nausea and vomiting can be common among children, especially teenagers who are undergoing cancer treatment, it pays to be aware of some of the things that can trigger it. Chelsea comments that an empty stomach can make them feel worse, so eating small amounts often is a good idea.

'Smells are important, and while not everyone will react it's better to keep children protected from strong smells; even things like perfumes and candles can be too much for some children. I don't wear perfume to hospital for this reason and because I've actually heard children telling a nurse to stay away as their perfume was making them feel sick.

'We already know that when you are unwell, some smells can be exaggerated, but there may be some scents, such as menthol and peppermint that can be good. Lemon, too – they're all fresh, clean smells.'

Children and adults often go off eggs, even in salads and cooking, says Chelsea, which can be a really big deal for them. Fish can also be a problem, but she's known people to still eat these foods, even if they think they have a problem with them, just as long as they are not exposed to the cooking smells. She cites an example where a child told her they didn't like eggs but there they were eating them. For this reason she believes it's often the smell, rather than the food itself.

As for the reason behind teenagers being particularly prone to nausea, Chelsea has observed that it can come from a place of anxiety.

'It's common for teenagers to walk through the doors to have their chemo and vomit before they are even hooked

up. It's a mind thing, which is hard to deal with. Distraction can be good in this situation; music and videos can focus their mind on other things. Some of them never think about how they might handle it while others fully embrace a strategy like choosing a song or songs to play in advance. Sometimes teenagers don't like to see the chemo apparatus, in which case we put a cover over it. It's all in the mind. Another example is the sight of a needle which for many people is no big deal but can result in terrible mind games for others.'

PAIN AND DISCOMFORT

'Deep breathing is very underrated as it can do a lot to reduce pain. Sometimes when I'm sitting with a child I can get them to breathe deeply by talking them through it, which will make them feel better. It takes a lot of concentration on their part, and it takes a little bit of confidence too.

'Distraction of one kind or another is good, especially when we have to give a child an injection. Although we try to do as much as we can through the drip, we can't always use it, so distracting them from what we're doing is a good strategy.

'Patting the area around the injection site stimulates the nerves, so helps it be less painful. We also use heat packs and cold packs, depending on the situation, to help ease pain.

'Then, of course, there are drugs for pain relief, but they tend to come with other side effects. Effective communication is key so we can maintain appropriate doses to ensure the medication is working. It depends on their age, but some children, usually seven or older, are quite capable of rating their pain on a scale of 1 to 10. But it can be hard for some children, no matter what their age.'

SIBLINGS

It's important for parents to take time to consider how any siblings might be feeling, and not just the ill child. Chelsea emphasises that it is such a big journey for everyone concerned.

'I feel for the siblings. Much depends on their age, but it can be hard on them seeing their sick sister or brother being allowed things that they're not permitted, such as treats to encourage them to put on weight. It's difficult for the other children to understand that it is only happening because the sibling is unwell.'

'If you think they are of an age to understand what is going on, then explaining to them why this is happening is probably a good idea. Tell them that their sister or brother is unwell, and so the normal rules have to be changed at this time. Explain that you understand why they think it is unfair, but that it's necessary to help get their brother or sister well again. Be clear that the child understands he or she is still much loved, even though so much attention is going to the sick one. And have this conversation, or variations on it, regularly. Also try to do something special with the well child, even if it is not as often as you'd like, away from the sick child. At such times keep the conversation away from the sick child and aspects of their sickness. Regular cuddles are also good as being close like this will reassure them.'

Sometimes while it might appear the sibling is coping really well with the situation, there might be more going on for them than is apparent. It's possible for them to get to a point where they will just snap because they feel things are so unfair. Be aware they will still need the same care and attention that you would give to a child who was clearly not doing well. In the case of two siblings, one could be doing great while the other is having difficulties. Just be sure to look after the one who seems to be doing great as well as the other one.

HAIR LOSS

Parents can sometimes be more upset about hair loss than the affected child. Obviously small children are unlikely even to notice while girls of four or five can get a bit upset. But in Chelsea's experience, this can be a result of how the parents have reacted. Teenagers vary in how they react, too – some of them are fine about it, while others freak out. Generally, though, children don't think too much about it – it is just one thing among many that they are having to cope with. They might wear beanies, although a lot of children find them uncomfortable. As a whole, it's usually not as upsetting as it can be for adults, who often have to be out in the world working and interacting with others in between treatments, making it a case of different dynamics.

EMOTIONAL WELLBEING

'Everyone, including kids, reacts differently on an emotional level. Some kids find writing or art therapy to be helpful in dealing with their feelings. But often it is just a matter of ensuring that they can do things they enjoy and keep busy when they can' – Chelsea

'It's important for their mind to stay occupied, which is where school work can come in. It's not so much for academic advantage but to help them to feel more

normal about their lives. Having little projects is good, and wherever possible let them pursue their previous interests. Reading, playing games, keeping busy with arts and craft, and seeing their friends are all positive things for them to do.

'It is particularly hard for the kids who are sporty, but there is nothing you can do about that. It's just tough. But sometimes it helps for them to watch their sport on TV and get enjoyment out of following a team. At least they are keeping up with it.

'It's also important for them to keep in touch with their sports teams, classmates, and other groups. A variety of photos is good, and you can stick these on the wall, especially if they are in the same hospital room for months. It's not always appropriate for their friends to visit, especially with the risk of infection, but Skype calls can work well. Technology can be great for sick children to keep in touch with their friends and classmates.'

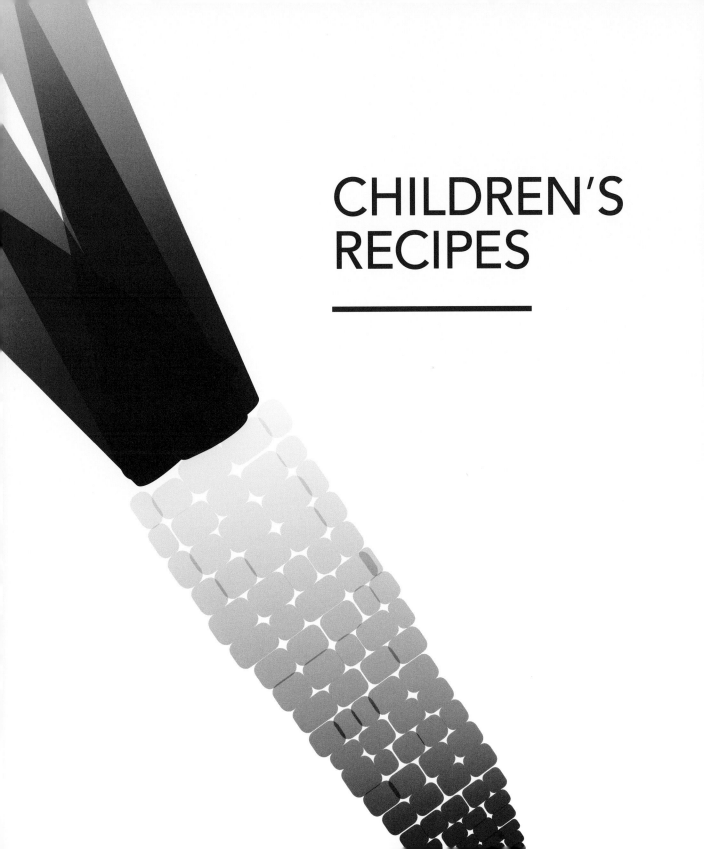

CHILDREN'S
RECIPES

Crepes

4–6   PREP: 5 min   COOKING TIME: a few minutes for each crepe

INGREDIENTS:

110g **flour**

pinch of **salt**

2 **eggs**

200ml **milk**

70ml **water**

50g (1.7oz) **butter**

Sift the flour and salt into a bowl. Make a well in the centre, drop in the eggs and whisk into the flour. Combine the milk and the water and add gradually into the mixture as you whisk. Melt the butter, add a third to the mix and stir in. Heat a shallow 20cm pan over a medium-high heat. Dip a scrunched up bit of paper towel into the remaining melted butter and grease the pan. Add a ladleful of batter and swirl to cover the base of the pan. Cook quickly on one side, lift the edge with a knife or palette knife, and flip over. The other side won't need any more than twenty seconds, then remove to a hot plate. Repeat until you are out of batter.

Sam: This standard recipe for both sweet and savoury crepes is something you will use constantly.

Karen: So simple to make, and a dish children will love! For this and any of the following recipes, if you can, cook the food away from children who are unwell.

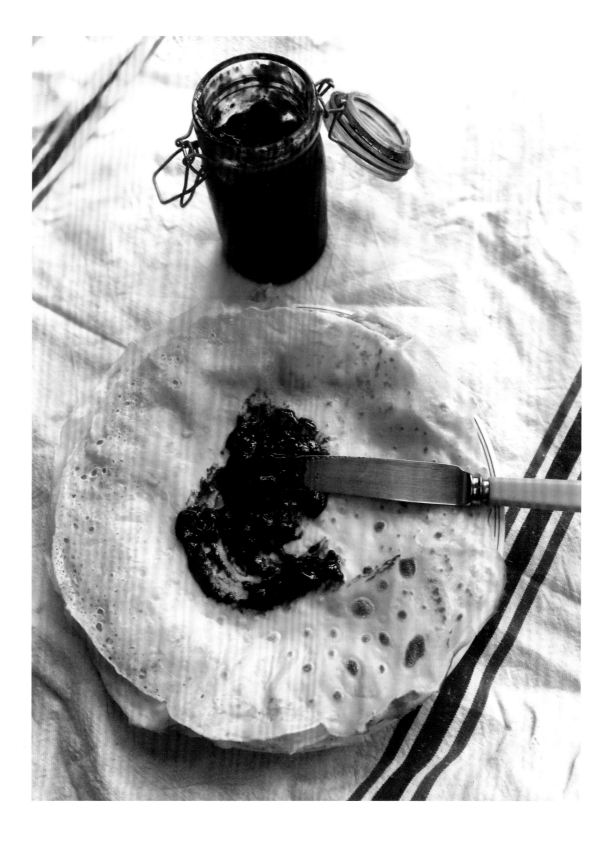

Sausage Rolls

4–6   PREP: 15 min   COOKING TIME: 40 min

INGREDIENTS:

50g (1.7oz) **butter**

1 **onion**, peeled and diced

4 cloves **garlic**, finely chopped

1 **bay leaf**

5 rashers of **bacon**, chopped
(shoulder or streaky)

2 tbsp **tomato paste**

50g (1.7oz) **fresh breadcrumbs**

several sprigs each of **rosemary**,
parsley and **thyme**, finely chopped

500g (17oz) **pork mince**

1 tsp **Dijon mustard**

2 **eggs**

salt and **pepper**

400g (14.1oz) packet of **puff pastry**

2 tbsp **sesame seeds**

In a frying pan over a moderate heat, add the butter and let it melt and bubble up. Add the chopped onion and garlic and fry gently for 3–4 minutes until it is soft and translucent. Add the bay leaf and chopped bacon and continue to cook gently until the bacon is starting to crisp. Add the tomato paste and let it cook and darken a little for several minutes, then remove the mixture from the pan to a large mixing bowl and leave to cool down for 5 minutes or so. Remove bay leaf. Add the breadcrumbs, chopped herbs, pork mince, Dijon, one of the eggs and a generous amount of salt and pepper and mix everything together well – your hands are best for this. Fry a little bit of the mixture off in the pan to taste and check if it needs any more seasoning.

Preheat the oven to 180°C on fan bake.

Take the pastry and roll out to a thickness of a couple of millimetres. Cut long rectangles about 15cm wide and run a 4–5cm wide length of the pork mixture down the middle. Beat the remaining egg and use to brush the pastry edges, then carefully roll the entire thing up into a log, pressing the edges down to seal them together. Cut into 6cm-ish lengths and place onto a lined baking tray. Make several slashes in the pastry on the top of each sausage roll, brush with beaten egg and then sprinkle the sesame seeds on top. Allow to bake for about 35–40 minutes, until the pastry is puffed and golden brown and the rolls are cooked through. Serve with a good tomato or plum sauce.

Karen: Cooked from scratch, children will love these sausage rolls, and you will have the satisfaction of knowing they are also nutritious and not full of any nasty additives.

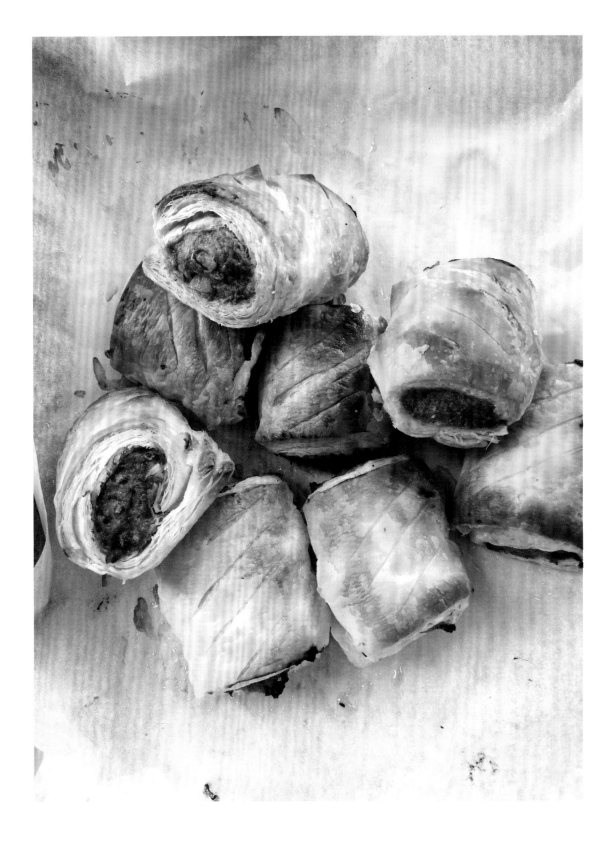

Hasselback Potatoes

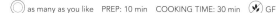 as many as you like   PREP: 10 min   COOKING TIME: 30 min   GF

INGREDIENTS:

waxy potatoes, such as new Agria or Jersey Benne

olive oil

salt and **pepper**

your favourite **cheese**

fresh **oregano**, **rosemary** or **thyme**

Preheat the oven to 180°C on fan bake.

Scrub the potatoes. Using a sharp paring knife, make multiple cuts about halfway down into each potato. Place on a lined baking tray and drizzle some olive oil over the potatoes. Season well and allow to bake for about 25–30 minutes, until they have puffed out and are crisp and golden. Remove from the oven and grate a generous amount of cheese over the top of them, pushing it down gently into the cuts, so that it will melt right through the potato. Scatter over a little bit of fresh herb and pop back into the oven for the cheese to melt down into the potatoes and go a little golden brown.

Karen: Children will love these tasty hasselback potatoes! It's the perfect comfort food when feeling unwell.

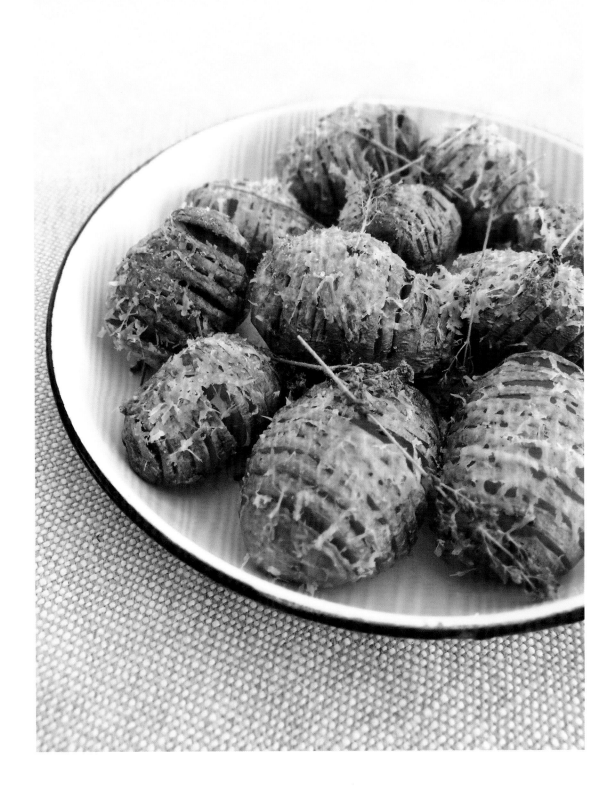

Grilled Whole Sweetcorn with Paprika and Cumin

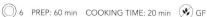 6   PREP: 60 min   COOKING TIME: 20 min   GF

INGREDIENTS:

6 whole **sweetcorn**, unhusked

3 tbsp **mayonnaise** or **aioli**

1 tsp **sweet paprika**

1 tsp **cumin seeds**

zest and **juice** of ½ **lemon**

salt and **pepper**

good **parmesan**, to serve

Pull the husks back from the sweetcorn, but don't remove them, so that they have handles for when time comes to eat them. Remove and discard the silk threads. Soak the corn in a sink or container of cold water for about an hour. Remove and shake off any excess water.

Get a lidded pot large enough to fit the corn, fill with hot water and bring to a gentle simmer over a medium heat. Add the corn and cook for about ten minutes. Drain and allow to cool a bit.

In a small bowl, combine the mayo, paprika, cumin, lemon zest and juice, and a bit of salt and pepper and combine well. Using your hands, use this mixture to smear well into the sweetcorn. Cover liberally with the mixture.

Get the barbecue or a hot grill going over a high heat. Place the sweetcorn down on the grill and cook on all sides for about 6–7 minutes until it is well caramelised all over. Remove from the heat and transfer to a serving platter and finely grate a generous amount of parmesan over the top. Serve immediately.

Karen: Corn is rich in nutrients, including the antioxidants beta-carotene and lutein, the carotenoids which give corn its distinctive colour. But of course, children will eat this just because this corn is simply delicious!

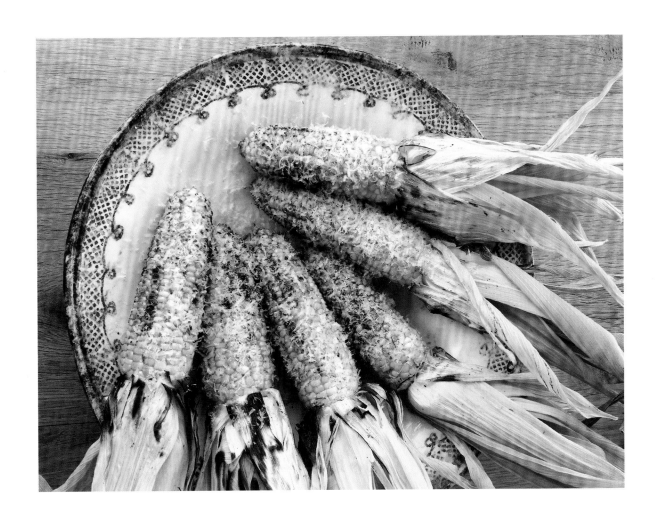

Jam Tarts

4–6   PREP: 30 min   COOKING TIME: 20 min

INGREDIENTS:

sweet shortcrust or **puff pastry**

your favourite **jam**

golden caster sugar

1 **lemon**

ice cream or **whipped cream**, to serve

Preheat the oven to 180°C on bake function.

On a clean, lightly floured bench, cut out rounds of pastry using a saucer – I like to use a 14cm diameter saucer. Blob a generous tablespoon of your favourite jam into each one and spread into a circle, leaving about 2cm of pastry showing on the edges. Fold the edges over about 3cm towards the middle, pinching the pastry together, and place the tarts onto an oven tray lined with baking paper. Pop them into the fridge for 25 minutes for the pastry to firm up, then sprinkle with golden caster sugar and bake for about 15–20 minutes, until golden brown. Zest the lemon over the top and serve alongside ice cream or whipped cream.

Karen: This is the perfect treat if you are worried about keeping your child's calories up, and they are very easy to make.

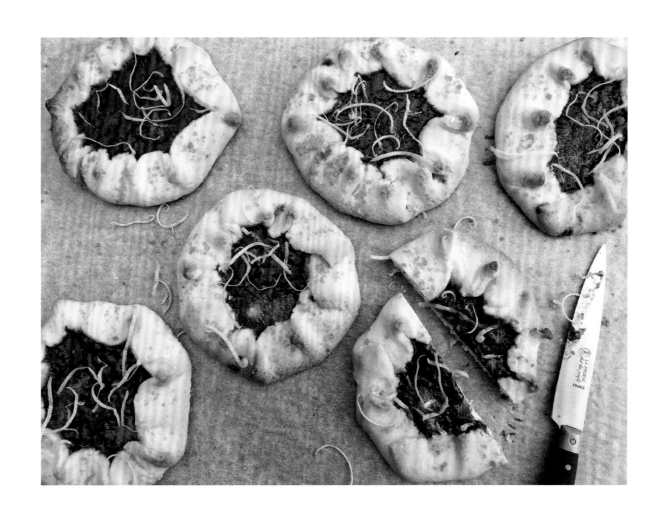

Panko Fish Bites

4-6   PREP: 120 min   COOKING TIME: 10 min in batches

INGREDIENTS:

500g (17.6oz) **firm white fish**, such as cod, gurnard, snapper or groper

½ cup (125ml) **coconut milk**

juice from 1 **lime**

1 tsp **sesame oil**

2 tsp **soy sauce**

1 **egg**, beaten

2 cups **panko crumbs**

salt and **pepper**

butter and **vegetable oil**, for frying

Cut the fish into bite sized pieces, about 6cm x 2cm, and place into a bowl. Combine with the coconut milk, lime juice, sesame oil and soy sauce and mix everything together well. Cover with cling film and leave to marinate in the fridge for at least two hours.

Remove from the fridge. Add the beaten egg to the fish so that the pieces are coated in the mix. Sprinkle the panko crumbs out on a plate, season with salt and pepper, and roll the fish pieces one by one in the crumbs to coat them on all sides.

Bring a frying pan up to a moderate heat. Add a teaspoon of butter and a little oil and let it melt and bubble up before frying the fish in batches until golden brown on all sides. Remove to kitchen paper to drain before serving with aioli or tartare sauce.

Karen: Fish is loaded with nutrients, but in particular it is the best source of omega-3 fatty acids, which are incredibly important for your body and brain.

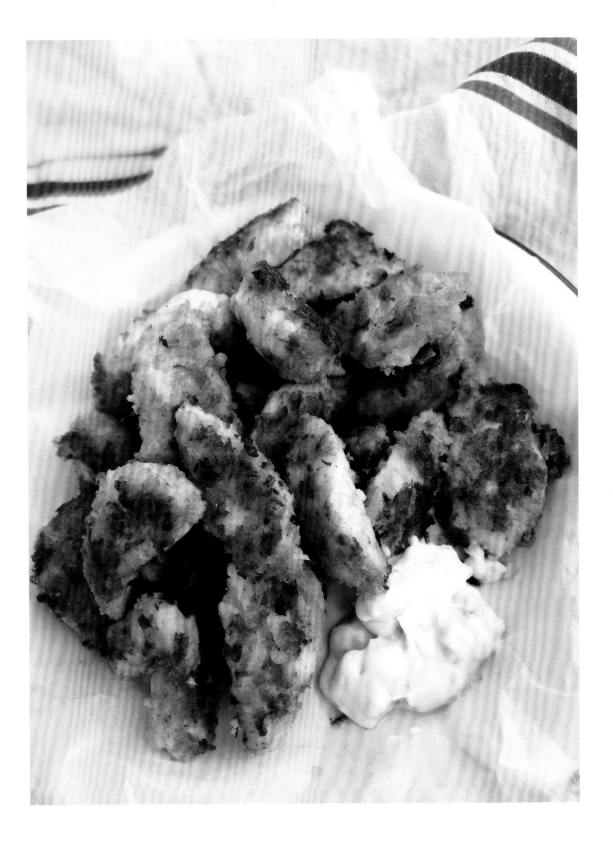

Courgette Pasta with Cream and Basil

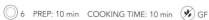 6   PREP: 10 min   COOKING TIME: 10 min   🌱 GF

INGREDIENTS:

6 **courgettes**

half a **lemon**

olive oil

salt and **pepper**

1 tbsp **butter**

200ml **cream**

large handful of **basil leaves**

parmesan, to serve

Wash and end the courgettes.

Using a julienne peeler, peel the courgettes into long thin strands. Transfer to a bowl, zest in the lemon and add a squeeze of juice, followed by a tablespoon of olive oil and some salt and pepper, and toss through.

In a saucepan over a moderate heat, add the butter and let it melt and bubble up. Follow with the cream, half the basil, and lots of salt and pepper, and let the cream bubble up, reduce down and thicken for several minutes. Fold in the courgette and let it warm through. Taste and season accordingly, then fold in the remaining basil and serve with generous gratings of parmesan over the top.

Karen: Courgettes, which are better known in some countries as zucchini, are full of vitamins and fibre. This is a 'pasta' dish that packs a nutritional punch.

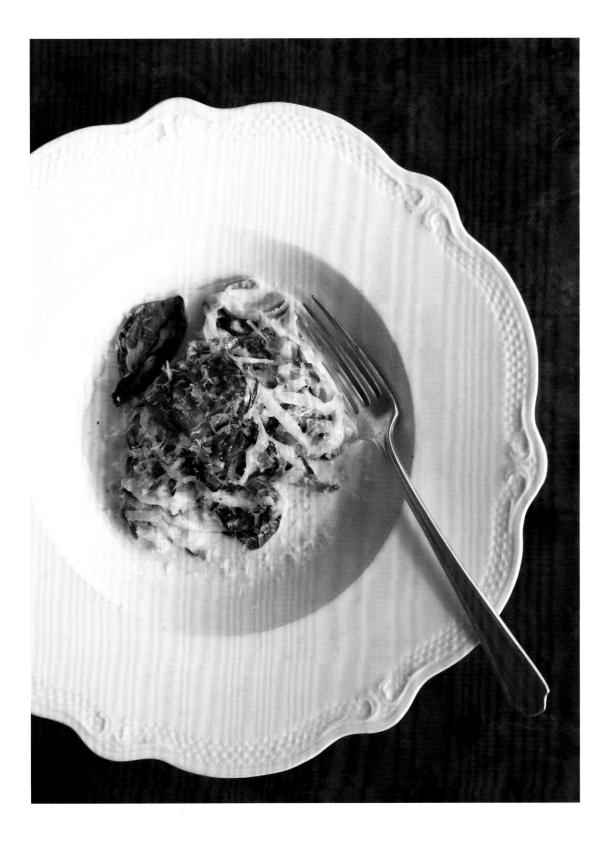

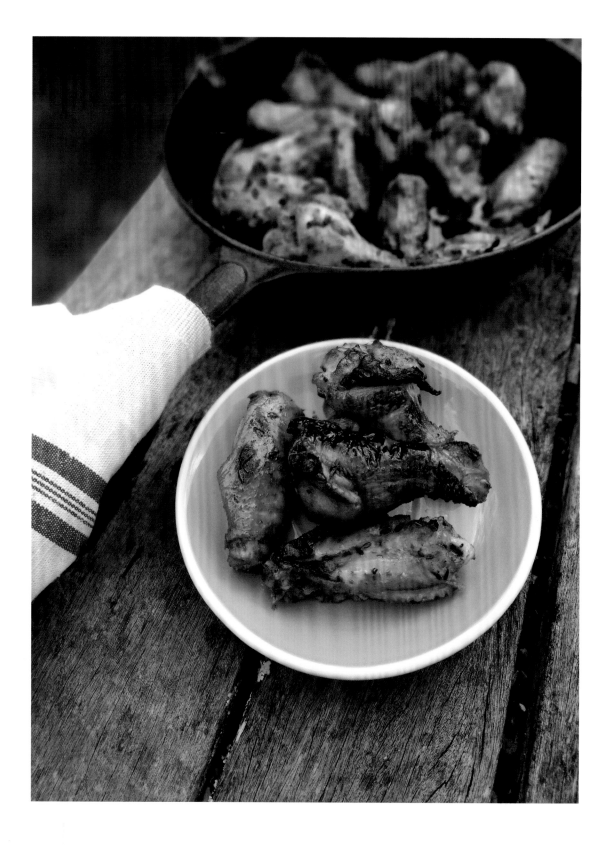

Chicken Nibbles with Soy and Honey

4–6   PREP: 120 min   COOKING TIME: 35 min   DF

INGREDIENTS:

1 kg (35oz) **chicken nibbles**

3 tbsp **light soy sauce**

2 tbsp **dark soy sauce**

3 tsp **runny honey**

1 tsp **cumin seeds**

Combine all ingredients thoroughly in a bowl. Cover with cling film and pop into the fridge to marinate for at least two hours.

Preheat the oven to 180°C on fan grill.

Remove the marinated nibbles from the fridge and transfer to an oiled roasting tray, spreading them out evenly. Roast for about 30–35 minutes, shaking them around occasionally so that they are cooked evenly on all sides, until the chicken is cooked through, golden brown and sticky. Allow to cool a little before serving.

Karen: For many people soy is a flavour that is appealing when going through cancer treatments, when other food tastes bland – and this recipe that Sam has created is particularly moreish!

Recipe Index

Acknowledgements

Thank you Sally Greer and Kitki Tong, both of Beatnik Publishing, for your support of this project and for producing such a beautiful book.

Thanks also to all the experts who feature in these pages. Your knowledge in your particular field has been invaluable in creating this book. And thanks to all the 'regular' people, for telling it how it is and sharing your insight.

Huge gratitude to oncologist Dr Reuben Broom for his encouragement, suggestions and guidance in this project. And special thanks to Dr Janice Brown for her invaluable help in the creation of this book also.

Sam: Mum and Dad – as always, thank you for your constant love, support and everything else in between.

Karen: A special thank you to my amazing husband, Iain McKenzie, for his love and ongoing support.

About the Authors

Karen McMillan is the author of both fiction and non-fiction books. Her non-fiction titles include *Unbreakable Spirit: Facing the Challenge of Cancer*, *Love Bytes*, *Feast or Famine: a New Zealand guide to understanding eating disorders*, *Unleash Your Inner Seductress*, and *From the Blitz to the Burmese Jungle and Beyond*, a World War II memoir. She has adapted *Dying: A New Zealand Guide to the Journey*, a South African book about dying for the local market, and her novels include *Brushstrokes of Memory*, *Watching Over Me*, and two historical novels, *The Paris of the East* and *The Paris of the West*.

Karen lives in Auckland, New Zealand, where she has volunteered for hospice for many years. You can read more about her at www.karenm.co.nz.

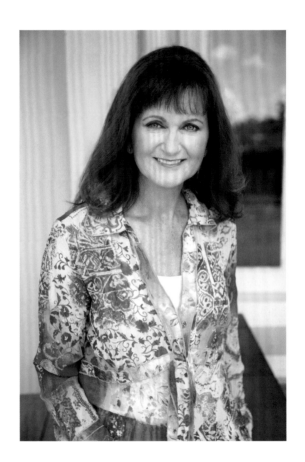

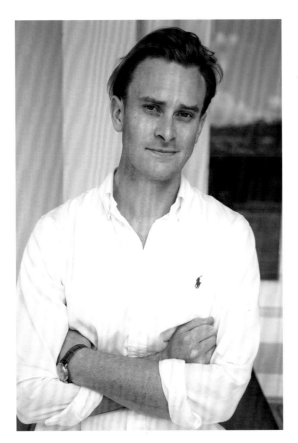

Sam Mannering is the author of the bestselling books *Food Worth Making* and *A Year's Worth: Recipes from Dunsandel Store*. He cooks, writes about food, and sometimes acts a bit, too. He studied at the Royal Central School of Speech and Drama in London.

He is the weekly food columnist in the *Sunday Star-Times*, and is a contributor to *Cuisine*, *House & Garden* and *UNO* magazine. He is the executive chef and co-owner of Homestead Eatery in Auckland.

A member of the board of the Wallace Arts Trust, since 2014 he has also been an ambassador for Totara Hospice, for Fisher & Paykel and for Cloudy Bay Wines.

Sam lives in Auckland, New Zealand. You can read more about him at www.sammannering.com.

Additional Information

For more information about some of the
experts, products or organisations from this
book, and other useful websites go to:

www.cancer.org

www.cancer.org.au

www.cancernz.org.nz

www.holistichair.co.nz

www.jessicaswigsalon.co.nz

www.macmillan.org.uk

www.megandempsey.co.nz

www.menopause.org.au

www.optimumhealth.co.nz

www.orasoothe.com

www.pincandsteel.com

www.prostate.org.nz

www.sweetlouise.co.nz

www.thewellernetwork.com